Musings

of a

Vermont Nutritionist

A *to* Z

Antioxidants *to* Zinc

Stories to Improve Your Health

by
Lyn Carew, PhD.

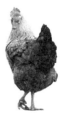

Published by Wind Ridge Publishing, Inc.
Partnership Books Division
P.O.Box 752
Shelburne, Vermont 05482

ISBN Number 978-1-935922-01-8

Library of Congress Control Number: 2010940235

Cover and Book Design by Laurie Thomas
Printed at Queen City Printers, Burlington, Vt., U.S.A.

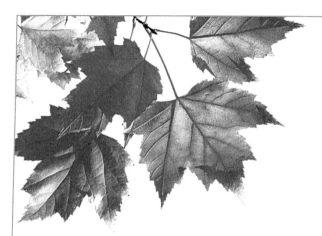

Musings of a Vermont Nutritionist

A *to* Z

Antioxidants to Zinc

Stories to Improve Your Health
by **Lyn Carew**, PhD.

Published by Wind Ridge Publishing, Inc.
Shelburne, Vermont

Contents

Healthy Holidays

Preface

Nutrition is fascinating. It involves almost all aspects of life: science, health, history, economics, politics, sociology, and more. Every story about nutrition has an interesting factual twist as well as a humorous one, or at least a curious one. After teaching human nutrition to thousands of students for more than forty years, the need for such illustrative nutrition stories occurred to me over and over again. When I put them into short articles for the local press, the enthusiastic response was unexpected.

Good nutrition is not all that complicated, and after reading the research literature daily, the old concept of a balanced, natural diet kept surfacing as the most reasonable approach, with a few caveats. For example, recent discoveries point to the health effects of larger amounts of vitamin D and omega-3 fatty acids than might be found in a balanced diet, and this requires more than just eating well. And there are some potential medical uses of unnaturally high doses of food components such as the antioxidant lutein, the B vitamin, niacin, and some others. In general, good nutritional health requires use of a natural, mainly unrefined food pattern with a fair amount of vegetables and fruits, coupled with some protein sources, some fat sources, and adequate minerals such as calcium. Diversity and a range of colorful foods are key. The main culprit in nutritional ill health is obesity, or eating too much of anything. Extreme diets are to be avoided. And of course, there is a need for exercise: humans evolved to run – either after something or away from something.

I intended these stories to give some commonsense to nutrition and health. And also some fun. That was my experience as I researched and wrote these stories, and it's my pleasure to introduce these nutritional musings to you.

Lyn Carew

Acknowledgements

I've been fortunate. For 42 years, many of my happiest moments have been in the classroom although I greatly enjoy research too. My thanks is offered to my students for providing the stimulus to write these illustrative nutritional stories in response to their many good questions and challenges. They kept me on my toes and made me be sure of what was in the scientific literature. Thanks to Margo Callaghan, the editor of Shelburne News at Wind Ridge Publishing (WRP), for initially encouraging me to put these ideas into print in monthly columns. Thanks to Holly Johnson, WRP publisher, whose support made this book possible, and to Lin Stone, WRP Partnership Books editor, whose significant suggestions helped get the articles into shape. I am indebted to fellow nutritionist and colleague, Deborah Paradis for help with the original editing, and who often served as Devil's Advocate to my ideas; her assistance was superb. Thanks to Dr. David Elvin, fellow biologist and colleague, whose computer expertise for over 30 years was invaluable in developing my teaching techniques. I have also been fortunate over the many years to be surrounded by a lifelong array of family, friends, colleagues, and neighbors, national and international, nearby and far away, who have been supportive and have made life enjoyable and interesting. I don't think you know how much you have all meant to me. Finally, but not least, I owe much to my best friend, Alida Ingham Lund, whose patience allowed me to be impatient at times as I accumulated the information found in this book.

Note to Readers

In these Musings, I use *kilocalories* when referring to the energy content of foods. This is the proper designation and although in the popular press the term calorie is used, that is not scientifically correct. An apple actually has 70 kilocalories, or 70,000 (small) calories, not 70 calories. My students would want it this way.

The information in this book is not designed to prevent, diagnose, or treat medical problems. It is intended for educational purposes only.

This book is dedicated to the loves of my life
~ my daughters, Leslie and Audre.

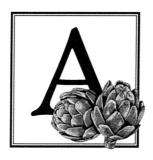

Anti-Oxidants
What Are They Against?

Antioxidant is a widely used buzzword in nutrition these days. Purveyors of foods, vitamin supplements, and even shampoos promote antioxidants. In the popular press, antioxidants are touted to prevent cancer and heart disease, and especially to slow aging. Take antioxidants and live longer? Should you keep antioxidant pills in your pocket and take several every day?

The "oxidant" part of antioxidant refers to the action of oxygen. We all know that we have to breathe oxygen in order to stay alive. Oxygen combines with fats and sugars in our body's cells to produce energy – the fats and sugars are "oxidized." That is good – that's what oxygen is designed to do. The problem arises when oxygen leaks out to parts of our cells where it shouldn't be. When this happens, the oxygen in the form of "free radicals" severely damages the body's tissues. Yes, oxygen is both good and bad.

To prevent damage from occurring, our cells contain antioxidants that can attach to this misplaced oxygen and carry it off or convert it to harmless water. But the catch here is that these antioxidants mostly come from foods. Some are well known such as vitamins E, C, and beta-carotene, and minerals such as selenium and zinc. But most are unknown and there are likely thousands of undiscovered antioxidants in foods that work by yet undiscovered mechanisms. The total antioxidant capacity of foods can be measured and is expressed in Oxygen Radical Absorbance Capacity (ORAC) units. Most fruits, vegetables, and whole grains contain substantial ORAC units, but blueberries, blackberries, and similar fruits, as well as vegetables such as artichokes and spinach, contain the most. Pinto and other beans are also loaded with antioxidants.

A problem arises when scientists try to isolate antioxidants from foods and put them in pills. When a high intake of tomatoes in Italian men was linked with prevention of prostate cancer, the red-colored antioxidant lycopene was isolated from tomatoes and sold in pills, but it didn't work. The consumption of red wine seemed to be the reason the French do not get a lot of heart disease in spite of eating lots of cream and cheese. Resveratrol, another antioxidant with another strange name, was isolated from wine but it has not been shown to reduce heart disease.

Dark colors in foods are definitely associated with high ORAC values, and recently, purple-colored antioxidants, known chemically as anthocyanins, were isolated from fruits and found to improve brain function. However, foods contain hundreds of anthocyanins and there is great doubt they work alone. On the other hand, strong evidence shows that whole foods, high in ORAC units, like blueberries, strawberries, and spinach, reverse brain aging in rats. One bright spot is the Age-related Eye Disease Study (AREDS); research shows that mixtures of individual antioxidants might help prevent macular degeneration, a disease that causes blindness in older people. But maybe eating foods that contain these antioxidants would work better. It's still being tested.

The important lesson here is that antioxidants most likely work in combination with other components in foods and do not work alone. The old-fashioned idea to eat lots of fruits and vegetables and stay away from refined foods works even better with antioxidants. So, antioxidants in whole foods work for you, not against you; they keep you healthy and perhaps help you to live longer.

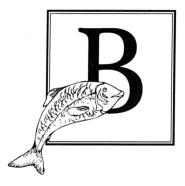

Brain Food
Is Fish Really That?

Was grandmother right when she said "Fish is brain food?" You remember her saying that, don't you? This notion has been around for generations. But what did it really mean? Fish is an excellent food, loaded with high-quality protein, and fair amounts of vitamins and minerals. In that way, it isn't much different from milk, soybeans, or meat. And certainly a fish doesn't resemble a brain any more than these other foods do. How then did fish gain this reputation?

This idea didn't make much sense to nutritionists. Fish meat is mainly muscle, and muscle has about 20 percent protein; brain is not muscle and has only 8 percent protein. Muscle has 5 percent lipids but brain has 12 percent, and a lot of that is cholesterol – much more than in fish, meat, and milk. Where could such a nonsensical idea have come from? Now, based on recent scientific evidence, grandma was right: eating fish can dramatically improve brain function.

Back in the 1970s, it was discovered that fish, especially ocean fish, contain fatty acids that are quite different from those found in most other foods such as vegetable oils, meat, and milk. Fish fatty acids are larger (contain more carbon atoms) and are more unsaturated (contain more double bonds). Fish oil fatty acids are frequently called omega-3s because one of the double bonds is three steps from the end, or omega part, of the fatty acid (omega means end in Greek) . These unique omega-3 fatty acids in fish are named docosahexaenoic acid and eicosapentaenoic acid, but who can remember that? So, they are referred to as DHA and EPA. It's important to recognize that these come almost exclusively from certain fish, and if you don't eat those fish your body may be deficient in them.

Since the 1970s, it's been established that omega-3 fatty acids from fish are essential for heart function. It's now highly recommended that you get two-three servings of ocean fish each week to reduce the risk of heart disease (or take fish oil or algae pills). This evidence is strong. These studies explain why Eskimos almost never had heart disease; their diet was loaded with fish.

More recently, it has been found that omega-3 fish oils also play a very important role in the structure and function of the brain. They thus affect thought processes and emotions. Such studies have shown that brain development in babies and subsequent performance of children in school are affected by the amounts of EPA and DHA in their diet. These results have been so revealing that many infant formulas now have EPA and DHA added to them. Look the next time you are in a store. Earlier infant formulas made from ingredients such as soybeans, and low-fat milk powder were probably deficient in omega-3 fatty acids, and this may partially explain why breast-fed babies were healthier than formula-fed babies were. Yes, it's possible, that prior to omega-3 supplementation of infant formulas, non-breast-fed babies were deficient in omega-3 fatty acids. Of equal importance is recent evidence suggesting that brain function in adults is also affected by omega-3 fatty acids in the diet. I had the honor of being invited to a conference in San Diego in which Commander Joseph Hibbeln, M.D., a nutritional psychiatrist with the U.S. Public Health Service, presented evidence showing that violent behavior in prison inmates may be related to low levels of omega-3 fatty acid in their blood. Beyond this there is some evidence that depression in adults and attention deficit disorder in children may be improved with omega-3 fatty acids, although this work is too early to rely on.

Based on such results, the American Psychiatric Association supported the following statement in the 2006 Journal of Clinical Psychiatry. I've abstracted it slightly.

"The preponderance of epidemiologic and tissue compositional studies supports a protective effect of omega-3 essential fatty acid intake, especially EPA and DHA from fish, on mood disorders."

So, besides eating fish to prevent heart disease, your psychological state may also depend on this food. The next time grandmother says, "fish is a brain food," ask her how she knew that before omega-3 fatty acids were discovered. And then send me the answer.

Omega-3 Fatty Acid Content of Some Fish gm/100gm

Anchovy	1.4
Bluefish	1.2
Halibut	0.9
Herring	1.6
Mackerel	2.5
Salmon	1.4
Sardines	5.0
Sturgeon	1.5
Tuna	1.6
Lake Trout	1.6
Rainbow Trout	0.5

Clams and most crustaceans such as shrimp, and lobster have only 0.2-0.5 gm/100gm.

Note: An omega-3 fatty acid is found in plants such as flaxseed and soybeans (called alpha linolenic acid, or ALA), but it is different from EPA and DHA in fish oil. To be active in the brain ALA must be converted to DHA and EPA. This conversion is very inefficient, about 10 percent, so plants are poor sources of "active" omega-3 fatty acids. Also, about 0.5-1 grams per day of fish omega-3s seems to be the required amount.

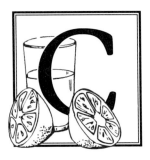

Vitamin C
Win, Place, Or Show?

People's interest in taking vitamins changes each year. It's similar to watching a horse race. Once vitamin C was in the lead. Now it's vitamin D with vitamin K close behind. Folic acid seems to be pulling up on the inside, but vitamin E is hanging back.

Over the years, vitamin C (aka ascorbic acid) has been the most popular vitamin that people purchase, but lately it's falling behind. Is it going to be a loser and wind up in last place? Let's look at the scientific information about this nutritional racehorse.

Vitamin C is one of the water-soluble vitamins. It is best known for the prevention of scurvy, a deficiency disease characterized by bleeding gums, pinpoint hemorrhages, and bruising in the skin. Historically, its deficiency led to the death of 60-70 percent of sailors in France, England, and other countries during exploratory days in the 1400-1700s. Deficiencies also occurred during the Civil War and World War I; they are still seen today among people who avoid fruits and vegetables and eat mainly grains, meat, and beans.

Vitamin C was the leading horse in the 1970s when it looked like high doses prevented colds. Dr. Linus Pauling, a world-renowned California Institute of Technology biochemist, claimed colds could be prevented with doses from 1,000 milligrams (mg)/day to 10,000-20,000 mg/day. The Recommended Daily Allowance (RDA) listed by the Institute of

Medicine is below 100 mg/day, so Dr. Pauling's suggested levels were massive. But, alas, he was wrong; there is little evidence that vitamin C prevents colds.

But this doesn't make vitamin C a loser. It is also a notable antioxidant (yes, like vitamin E) and as such it may play a role in preventing some major diseases like cancer and heart disease. The current recommended intake of vitamin C is 75 mg and 90 mg per day for adult women and men, respectively (as little as 10 mg/day will prevent scurvy). Some years ago, I heard an excellent seminar from Cornell in which it was indicated that about 200 mg/day are needed based on saturation of white blood cells with vitamin C. This meant that the body was still using vitamin C at this level and not excreting it. This research also showed that blood levels of vitamin C drop during stress such as hard physical activity, and at least 200 mg/day were needed to maintain proper saturation.

Vitamin C is one of the few nutrients that is definitely affected by stress. Its need seems to increase in heat stress and also during athletic activities. Recently, a report from Beloit College suggested that levels of 500 mg twice daily might be needed in situations of extreme stress such as war zones and traumatic brain injury. Also, there is evidence that vitamin C might help prevent macular degeneration, lower blood pressure, and slow the aging process as well. Certainly, it's known that stress imposed on the body by smoking increases the need for vitamin C by 35 mg/day.

Taken together, these results suggest we might aim for higher levels of vitamin C than suggested by the RDAs. You might want to somewhat increase your intake of orange juice (124 mg/cup), or add a variety of other fruits and vegetables such cranberry juice (107 mg/cup), broccoli (106 mg/stalk), and yellow sweet peppers (218 mg each, raw).

Who knows, all eyes may turn to look at this vitamin again. Some of the positive effects of vitamin C may not be unique and may be related to its antioxidant properties, which can possibly be replaced by antioxidants in other foods. We don't know that yet. And to reach intakes in the high range of 1,000 mg/day, a supplement might be needed, but let's not go there until the race is finished. It's clear that vitamin C is not a loser. Like its racehorse namesake, C-biscuit, vitamin C might just be waiting for its chance to charge ahead and take the lead once again. Just keep your eye on this horse and the finish line.

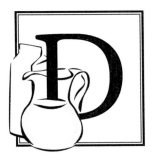

Vitamin D
It May Save Your Life

I hope I got your attention because vitamin D is one of the hottest and most important subjects in nutrition today. And you may be deficient, especially during Vermont's long winter months.

We've known for years that vitamin D promotes strong bones and prevents diseases such as rickets and osteomalacia in which bones become soft and bend. But recently, much fairly strong research has shown that getting adequate vitamin D may prevent several forms of cancer, including colon, prostate, breast, and pancreatic cancers. This is not a minor matter – paying attention may save your life. Vitamin D is quite different from other vitamins in that it is actually a hormone, and hormones have a diversity of actions in the body. Research shows that vitamin D can regulate and interfere with the very cellular processes that promote cancer. Beyond this, there is reasonable evidence that adequate vitamin D may prevent multiple sclerosis, gum disease, and hypertension, and a deficiency of vitamin D may play a role in heart disease, lupus, diabetes, osteoarthritis, osteoporosis, weakness in elderly, and several other problems, even the flu. Wow! Curiously, some diseases such as prostate cancer and multiple sclerosis are more prevalent in the higher latitudes as you move closer to the North Pole.

Vitamin D is produced by exposure of the skin to ultraviolet sunlight and is sometimes called the "sunshine vitamin." We get some through our diet, but plant foods are almost devoid of it. Animal sources such as fatty fish, eggs, and butter contain low levels that are usually not enough to meet your needs. Vitamin D synthesis from sunlight is almost essential!

Over a century ago, in cloudy northern cities like Burlington, Cleveland, and Seattle, more than 50 percent of children developed rickets in the winter. Since its discovery in the 1930s, vitamin D has been added to milk and the incidence of rickets has plummeted. However, a quart of milk supplies only 400 International Units (IU) of vitamin D, barely enough to help bones, but probably not enough to prevent the other diseases listed above. Many researchers, including Dr. Michael Hollick, a leading vitamin D researcher and director of the Bone Health Care Clinic at Boston University Medical Center, think that we should aim for a minimum of 1,000 IU a day. But the only food to supply that amount is a dose of cod liver oil (1,300 IU/tablespoon). A 4 oz. serving of salmon supplies 410 IU, a can of sardines 230 IU, an egg 25 IU, and a tablespoon of butter 8 IU. The vitamin D (D_2) in breakfast cereals is not used as readily as that in animal products (D_3). This leads to the recommendation that vitamin D supplements are frequently necessary. We still must be careful however, because the upper limit currently considered safe is 2,000 IU/day, although with more research it looks as though it could be set much higher than that. Some diseases, such as Parkinson's disease, have been reported to respond to much higher doses of vitamin D, but results are limited.

In Vermont, we may get enough vitamin D in the summer, but from November to March, the sun is so low in the sky that ultraviolet rays (UVB) responsible for vitamin D synthesis in the skin do not get through the atmosphere. And we may not be able to relax our concerns in the summer. A recent study from Hawaii indicates that in spite of abundant sunshine, vitamin D levels are still low in some inhabitants, even when skin color is taken into account (darker skins are less efficient at vitamin D synthesis). The risk of vitamin D deficiency increases with the use of sunscreens – up to a 95 percent reduction in vitamin D synthesis, and skin becomes less efficient at this task as we age.

As Vermont days shorten and the sun irrevocably moves south, we should enlighten ourselves: a vitamin D supplement may be necessary to sustain the sunniest of healthy lives.

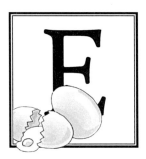

Eggs
Are They Really Bad?

You wouldn't want to be friends with bad eggs, especially if they cause heart disease. Think back over the last 30-40 years and perhaps you recall hearing, "eggs are loaded with cholesterol and can clog your arteries," "eat only two eggs a week," or "throw the yolk away and only eat the white." Do you remember that? These ideas were widespread in professional journals, textbooks, magazines, and newspapers. A group of top biological scientists I knew in the 1970s even promoted the idea of labeling all egg cartons like cigarettes, stating that they are unsafe for your health.

The bad news about eggs was related to their high cholesterol content. But to the contrary, there was not much evidence that eating egg yolk cholesterol increased the incidence of heart disease. Researchers who work with chickens and eggs have known that for many years. Yes, if someone has serious blood cholesterol issues then by all means follow a knowledgeable physician's advice to lower it, including not eating eggs. But for the vast majority of people, eggs do no harm. Cascades of false beliefs happen repeatedly in nutrition as well as in the rest of life. A startling and superficially logical statement will be repeated in articles and books without the diligence of questioning the original source. "Great is the power of steady misrepresentation," said Charles Darwin.

We now know that eating egg cholesterol does not increase blood cholesterol in harmful ways for most people. The two sources of cholesterol are not tightly linked. If eating eggs does slightly elevate blood cholesterol, the "good" HDL cholesterol goes up with the "bad" LDL, but most often, even if a dozen eggs is consumed, little happens to blood cholesterol because the body shuts off its manufacture of cholesterol.

A sad side of this story is that many people switched from eating eggs at breakfast to consuming sugary things such as cereals, donuts, Danish, and bagels, etc. And what damage that must have done to their health. We've known for decades that eggs contain lots of protein, vitamins, minerals, and essential fatty acids. Two eggs supply 12 grams of protein or 20-25 percent of your daily need, and the quality of egg protein tops the charts. Fortunately, this trend reversed and these great packets of nutrients are more common at breakfast. The news gets better. Two recent scientific studies show that eating eggs at breakfast helps with weight loss – they fight obesity! Why? Replacing two donuts at breakfast (300-400 kilocalories each) with two eggs (75 kilocalories each) gives one obvious answer. But also, protein is an appetite suppressant while sugar does just the opposite. And we all know that sugar in the morning makes us sleepy while protein keeps us peppy.

Eggs may also help prevent macular degeneration of our eyes as we age. Eggs are excellent sources of two pigments called lutein and zeaxanthin that function as part of our eyesight mechanism, but they disappear as macular degeneration progresses. Eating eggs elevates blood levels of these pigments even more than spinach. Another recent report revealed that eggs reduce tissue inflammation, which can be a major cause of common diseases such as cancer and atherosclerosis. Eggs can play a positive role in nutrition and health. So, consider inviting a couple of good eggs over for breakfast.

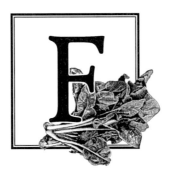

Folate
The Fickle Vitamin

F olate (or folic acid) isn't exactly a vitamin that's on the tip of every-one's tongue as are vitamin C or vitamin E. Yet it has come closest to being a magic bullet over the last two decades than has any vitamin. However, concerns with its use as a supplement have arisen.

Folate is one of the water-soluble B vitamins. It isn't called a B-anything like riboflavin, which is known as vitamin B-2; it's just folate. But folate goes by another name – folic acid. The important difference is that folate is the chemical form found in natural foods whereas folic acid is the chemical form used as a supplement in vitamin pills and cereals. They are closely related, but this distinction is very significant. Keep this in mind for our discussion later.

For years, folate was considered the vitamin most widely deficient in the U.S. diet because it is easily destroyed by heat, light, and oxidation. Also, it is mainly found in vegetables and beans, foods many people don't eat. A meat and potatoes diet is usually low in folate.

The main effect of a folate deficiency is a severe anemia accompanied by a sore, inflamed mouth and tongue. However, the almost miraculous news about folate over the last 30 years was that adequate intake just pri-or to and during pregnancy reduced the incidence of a tragic birth defect know as spina bifida by about 70 percent. This condition is a result of improper development of the nervous system. Due to this important role of folate, an FDA law was passed in 1996 mandating that folic acid (the artificial form of folate) be added to most grain products. Few people knew that this change had taken place.

Concern about this law has grown because experiments in animals suggest that in certain situations, mild supplements of folic acid could promote cancer; it made precancerous growths develop faster. These data were sufficiently worrisome that many European countries refused to allow supplementation of foods with folic acid. The greatest concern is for older people because cancer is an age-related disease.

Now the important twist. It appears that the artificial form called folic acid is the culprit and not folate found in foods. Why this might be so is not known, and the studies are so new that it might not even be true. I'm not sure why folate isn't used as the supplement instead of folic acid, but it is probably related to stability, cost, or availability. The lesson here, though, is not to take supplements with high amounts of folic acid in them.

This is a narrow line to walk because adequate folate/folic acid has a very positive side and has been reported to reduce heart disease, improve memory, reduce blood pressure, improve age-related hearing loss, reduce mental depression, and even prevent breast cancer.

What is the correct amount of folic acid to take? Nobody knows for sure, and certainly, during pregnancy a physician's advice should be followed. The Dietary Reference Intake by the Institute of Medicine is 400 micrograms (ug) per day (500-600 ug during lactation and pregnancy). Most vitamin pills supply 400 ug. The 1996 supplement law requires that 140 ug be added to each 100 grams of grain flour. Some suggest that 800-1,000 ug /day should be the upper limit especially for older people, but this is really an unknown number.

So at this point you have probably guessed the solution to this quandary – get your folate needs mainly from foods. Be wary of high supplements until this problem is resolved. But these concerns should not steer women of childbearing age away from proper supplements of folic acid. Even though it is fickle, folic acid produces some very good results.

Folate in Foods in micrograms

Lentils/black-eyed peas, ½ cup	179
Spinach, cooked, ½ cup	132
Black beans, cooked, ½ cup	128
Asparagus, cooked, ½ cup	122
Broccoli, cooked, ½ cup	84
Lettuce, ¼ of 6" head	75
Squash, winter, ½ cup	53
Orange juice, 1 cup	45
Potato, baked, 1	22
Apple or Peach, raw, 1	5

Beef liver, one of the few meats that contains much folate, has 260 ug/4 oz.

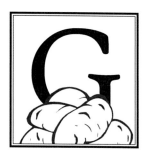

Glycemic Index
Stop Eating Potatoes?

Every now and then, new nutritional concepts come "blowin' in the wind" that profess to cure many problems. One of the latest is to stop eating potatoes because they increase the glycemic index, or GI. Stop eating potatoes? My gosh! When the Irish were forced to do this, they died! However, some of the country's best-known nutritionists have been fostering the idea that regulating the glycemic index can help to cure obesity, diabetes, heart disease, decreased physical performance, and a variety of other metabolic problems.

The glycemic index measures the rate that blood sugar rises after eating a meal: the faster sugar or starch is digested and absorbed, the higher the GI. Sometimes something called the glycemic load, or GL, is used to measure the total effect of a food on blood sugar level; they are both related. It is true that after eating a meal, rapid increases in blood sugar are accompanied by rapid increases in insulin, the hormone that regulates blood sugar. This can be followed by sharp deceases in blood sugar, which bring on feelings of fatigue and hunger. Sugary and processed foods tend to have a high GI. This is why it is not recommended to eat candy bars just before an athletic event or donuts for breakfast. You may feel peppy as blood sugar goes up quickly, but in an hour or two, the subsequent rapid fall in blood sugar can lead to tiredness and weak physical performance. It's better to have blood sugar rise more moderately.

Although it has been suggested that the concept of the glycemic index has application to people with diabetes, a recent issue of the highly respected American Journal of Clinical Nutrition contains three research articles showing that this may not be true.

A problem with the glycemic index is that it was developed by feeding people and animals single foods alone, such as potato, carrots, or bread, etc., and that is not the natural way we eat – we eat meals. The sugar, glucose (also called dextrose), is used as a standard of 100 when it is fed alone. This gives close to the maximum rise in blood sugar expected from any single food. By the same test, mashed potato with all its starch has a GI of 70-95, and beans, with all their digestion-slowing fiber and protein, have a GI of about 35. Because potato behaves like sugar, some say it should be avoided. However, potato is rarely eaten alone; more often it is eaten with fatty gravy or butter, which has little effect on the glycemic index and suppresses the GI of potatoes.

Curiously, ice cream has a low GI – shall we recommend that in place of potato? We might vote yes, but...hmm. We must remember that potatoes contain many essential minerals, and the skin has the best soluble fiber of any food. The glycemic index may be misleading and may be an eating guide that's too difficult to follow. So, perhaps we should keep potatoes on the plate and add a little gravy or butter to keep the glycemic index in check.

For now, the answer as to whether we should eat potatoes is stated best in Bob Dylan's song: "The answer my friend, is blowin' in the wind."

P.S. Visit www.mendosa.com for the GI list of hundreds of foods.

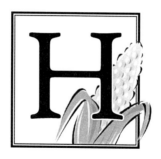

High Fructose Corn Syrup
Just The Facts, Ma'am

High fructose corn syrup (HFCS) appeared on the market about 1970. Since then it has received very bad press and has been blamed for many health problems, especially obesity and diabetes. Is this true? As Sgt. Joe Friday in the old TV series *Dragnet* might say, "We just want the facts, ma'am."

It's a fact that consumption of HFCS has increased markedly since 1970, while intake of regular table sugar has dropped. Now, per capita consumption of HFCS is about 60 lbs. per year and consumption of regular table sugar has dropped by half to 60 lbs. per year.

It's a fact that HFCS is not natural. It is produced by chemically altering the starch from the corn kernel. Natural table sugar or sucrose that you buy in a 5 lb. bag is extracted from sugar cane or sugar beets and consumed in that form. On the other hand, a convoluted process makes HFCS. First, the starch in corn kernels is extracted. Then it's treated with biological catalysts called enzymes. This converts the natural sugar glucose in the starch into another sugar called fructose. These two simple sugars, glucose and fructose, are then mixed together in an approximate 50/50 ratio. Actually, two mixtures of HFCS are used: 55 percent fructose/45 percent glucose in soft drinks and 42 percent fructose/58 percent glucose in baked goods.

It's a fact that HFCS closely resembles natural table sugar. Table sugar is a 50/50 mixture of glucose and fructose. It differs from HFCS in that table sugar's fructose and glucose are attached to each other whereas in HFCS they exist independently. This difference led some nutritionists to claim HFCS behaves differently in the body and causes health problems.

It's a fact that HFCS does not cause obesity, at least no more than over consumption of table sugar would. In 2004, one of the world's best obesity research laboratories reported a strong correlation between the rise in obesity since 1970 and increased intake of HFCS. This group claimed that HFCS was a major contributor to our growing waistlines. However, since then several scientific studies found no unique effect of HFCS on weight gain and the original researchers backed down on their claim.

It's a fact that some scientists have confused the situation by careless reporting. Because HFCS resembles table sugar, the two are usually handled in the body in similar ways. Unfortunately, some researchers have been feeding subjects large doses of fructose alone – not with its companion glucose. It's been known for some time that pure fructose, which we never encounter naturally in large amounts, is harmful and can elevate blood lipids and blood pressure among other effects. But when it's accompanied by similar amounts of glucose, it doesn't appear to act differently than table sugar. It's disturbing that no distinction was made between 100 percent fructose and HFCS. If you read that HFCS has harmful effects, find out if they really studied HFCS, or in fact, did they use pure fructose.

On the other hand, it's a fact that free fructose in HFCS could behave differently than the bound fructose in table sugar. One recent report suggested that cooking with HFCS produces harmful chemicals because the free fructose is chemically altered by heat. So HFCS is not out of the woods yet.

It's a fact that HFCS is not sweeter than table sugar. Yet some people claim they can detect differences between the two. As a result, some bakeries and soft drink companies are reverting to old-fashioned table sugar.

In the end, whether it's HFCS or table sugar, these are two "foods" not highly recommended as neither one has any nutritional value.

Well, those are the facts, ma'am. I hope Sgt. Friday found enough facts to close this case and not drag us off to the slammer.

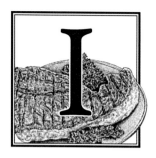

Iron
A Jekyll And Hyde Mineral

Iron is an essential mineral and iron supplements have probably done more good than any other nutrient. It is deficient in millions of people around the world – in women during their reproductive years due to the periodic loses of blood in the menstrual cycle and in young children. Yet like Dr. Jekyll in Robert Louis Stevenson's classic novel, it can change character and become very bad like Mr. Hyde.

Iron functions as part of the red hemoglobin within red blood cells. It helps transport oxygen from the lungs to all parts of the body, and this is necessary to sustain life. Iron deficiency produces anemia – a lack of the red hemoglobin in the blood. Red blood cells become small and pale, and oxygen cannot be distributed throughout the body and tissues. The oxygen we breathe is used to produce energy, so no wonder the greatest symptom of iron deficiency is fatigue.

Babies and other young mammals are very prone to iron-deficiency anemia because milk contains very little iron – milk isn't quite a perfect food. This is one reason why solid foods are started early for babies. Meats, with the obvious iron-containing red hemoglobin present, are the best source of iron. But iron in foods of plant origin is a different story. Although whole cereals, beans, legumes, and even a potato or apple have some iron, it is poorly available – much of it travels through the intestines unabsorbed.

Vegetarians thus have to pay special attention to sources of iron. While spinach contains lots of iron, almost none of it is absorbed because it is strongly attached to a chemical, oxalic acid, that won't let go of it in the intestine. However, combining these plant foods with acidic foods like orange juice can markedly increase the availability of iron. Some foods like broccoli contain both iron and vitamin C, and iron absorption is better here. Molasses is also a great source of iron for vegetarians.

But like Dr. Jekyll, iron has a strange side to it. While a little can do so much good, excess iron can kill you in the long run. One reason is that once in the body iron stays there permanently. It is not excreted in the urine and feces like other minerals. Iron is only excreted from the body by bleeding. Because of this it can build up in the tissues and destroy cells. Excess iron changes character and becomes a "pro-oxidant," just the opposite of all those good anti-oxidants we've discussed previously in this book. This means that overuse of iron could lead to heart disease and cancer.

People who continuously take high levels of iron put themselves in danger; they overload their body and this leads to tissue damage. While menstruating women lose iron regularly, once they reach menopause this stops and their need for iron drops dramatically. Nutritional supplements for seniors frequently omit iron entirely because not much is needed and it can be harmful to aging tissues. The misleading idea that if a little of a nutrient is good for you then a lot more is better definitely does not hold true for iron. So like the characters, Dr. Jekyll and Mr. Hyde in Stevenson's novel, at times iron is very nice, but at other times it can be very, very bad.

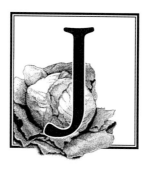

Joking Around
But Not With Cruciferous

You might think a nutritionist was joking with you if she said it would be a good idea to eat some cruciferous vegetables every day. The word sounds kind of tricky. Can you really buy cruciferous vegetables? This may sound funny, but don't stop reading or walk away – this is serious business.

What are cruciferous vegetables? Where do they come from? Are they good for you? You won't find a bin in the grocery store labeled "*Cruciferous*." But eating these vegetables may be one of the most important ways to maintain good health and especially reduce the risk of cancer.

Cruciferous vegetables are identified in a special way – they form the cabbage family. Included here along with cabbage are broccoli, cauliflower, turnip, rutabaga, Brussels sprouts, kohlrabi, bok choy, and kale, names that are familiar in the supermarket or the summer farmers' markets. Botanically they are in the *Brassicaceae* family but are often referred to as cruciferous because the flowers are arranged in a cluster of four that form a cross. More importantly, they contain unique substances that have been reported to significantly reduce the risk of cancer. Scientific data are sufficiently strong that groups like the National Cancer Institute recommend getting 1-2 serving of cruciferous vegetables every day.

Studies leading to these observations started years ago when it was observed that children in underdeveloped countries, deprived of sources of vitamin A (because they couldn't afford expensive vitamin A-containing foods such as eggs and butter) seemed to be at risk of developing various forms of cancer when they got older. This led nutritionists to compare sources of vitamin A itself with those in plants that contain the yellowish and orange pigment called beta-carotene, which is later converted to vitamin A in our intestines. These early investigations measured the degree of lung cancer in smokers. Surprisingly, when vitamin A was compared to carrots (a great source of beta-carotene), the cigarette smokers who ate the most carrots developed less lung cancer; carrots with their carotene appeared to be much more effective than vitamin A itself. This then led nutritionists to look at specific vegetables and the cruciferous vegetable group was found to be especially potent against cancer, but for another reason. Besides beta-carotene, these foods contain natural chemicals with strange names such as indoles and isothiocyanates that appear to strongly fight cancer, and these substances are not found in most other vegetables. That's why a serving or two daily from the cruciferous group is so important. But they should not be eaten to the exclusion of other vegetables, which may have their own beneficial chemicals such as antioxidants. Also, in large amounts, cruciferous vegetables can inhibit thyroid function, but you would have to eat an awful lot.

Cruciferous vegetables like most plants should not be cooked in boiling water because the beneficial substances are extracted into the cooking water. Although eating them raw isn't bad advice, mild cooking such as steaming or microwaving does not reduce the nutritional value.

So, don't be fooled by names; cruciferous vegetables are no joke. They also contain myriad nutrients that other vegetables have such as vitamin C, fiber, folic acid, potassium, and many others. In addition, they have their own beneficial chemicals that you should try to take advantage of each day. And we are not fooling you about this!

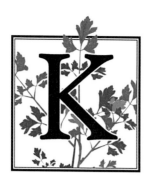

Vitamin K
A New Magic Bullet?

V itamin K has been a rather boring nutrient to discuss. For years, as far as we knew, it had only one function – to aid in the clotting of blood. If it was deficient, blood would not clot and extensive hemorrhaging would occur – even leading to death. Certainly, that was extremely important. But that was its sole function, and as important as this was, it wasn't very exciting to talk about and doing so put a damper on conversations. Especially so when compared to vitamin C and vitamin E, which were touted to prevent many different diseases, in addition to their own respective proprietary effects on scurvy and blood disorders.

Vitamin K is one of the four fat-soluble vitamins along with vitamins A, D, and E and is usually consumed in adequate quantities if one eats many leafy greens. Because vitamin K was so boring, it wasn't studied extensively in terms of human nutrition. This changed quickly over the last 10 years. In 1997, Dr. James Sadowski at Tufts University reported that vitamin K is also involved in bone health. This is well established now and the underlying biology is being studied extensively. Unlike calcium and phosphorus, which are necessary for the production of hard mineral in bone, vitamin K's role is in the synthesis of proteins in the soft part of bone.

People are often surprised to learn that only about half of bone structure is made up of mineral (called apatite), and most of the rest is made up of protein. If one were to remove the mineral from bone, it would retain its size, but what was left would be soft and rubbery like a dog's play bone; this would be mostly protein.

It was almost startling to nutritionists when the discovery about vitamin K and bone was followed by reports that Vitamin K had several other functions in the body. High levels of vitamin K may slow the development of heart disease by preventing the calcification and stiffening of coronary (heart) arteries. Wow! By this same mechanism, vitamin K may play a role in Alzheimer's disease. Wow again! As more investigators got on the vitamin K bandwagon, new reports suggested that it also prevented diabetes and liver cancer. And biochemists found that vitamin K acts as an antioxidant and may play an important role in reducing inflammation, which can be the leading cause of several important diseases. Thus, boring vitamin K became very exciting.

All of this new information does not mean that people should start taking vitamin K pills. To the contrary, vitamin K is a tricky vitamin. First, it occurs in several forms, and it is not known which form is most important in preventing certain diseases. Second, a lot of the research has been done in animals and so we must wait confirmation in humans. Third, a well-balanced diet high in green leafy vegetable supplies adequate amounts of vitamin K. Certainly, a fast food, or a meat and potatoes diet is not adequate. Animal products are low in vitamin K.

People on blood thinners such as coumadin (Warfarin) should not fool around with vitamin K. This can be very dangerous. Coumadin's main role is to alter vitamin K levels in the body. As a coumadin user myself, I will await new research and definitely follow my physician's advise.

So vitamin K is not exactly a new magic bullet, but it joins its fat-soluble cousins, A, D, and E in having several important roles in our health. Now when we hear about vitamin K, our ears should perk up to listen to all the new stuff coming down the research road. This also gives us good reason to pay attention to all those wonderful salad recipes that include lots of greens along with the meat and potatoes.

Vitamin K in Foods* micrograms/100 grams

Parsley, raw	1640
Kale, cooked	817
Spinach, raw	483
Collard greens, cooked	440
Swiss chard, cooked	327
Brussels sprouts	140
Broccoli, raw	102
Canola oil	71
Blueberries, canned	20
Tomato, raw	8
Butter	7
Liver, beef, braised	3
Tuna, canned	3
Milk, whole	1
Eggs, poached	0.3

Estimated need = 60-90 mcg/day
* USDA Nutrient Database

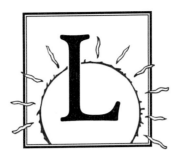

Licking The Flu!
Vitamin D Will Do

Take vitamin D and you might not get the flu! That might sound like science fiction, but evidence is slowly accumulating that vitamin D plays a role in a variety of diseases including the flu. For years it was thought that the childhood condition of soft, bending bones called rickets was the main symptom of a lack of vitamin D. Now, breast cancer, colon cancer, Type I diabetes, hypertension, falls in the elderly, and even obesity have been correlated with low blood levels of vitamin D. But for now let's focus on the flu.

When winter sets in, many Northerners face a vitamin D deficiency. Most vitamin D in our bodies is produced by ultraviolet sunlight falling on our skin (thus its nickname "the sunshine vitamin"). As the northern sun sets lower in the sky from November to March, very few ultraviolet rays reach us. Add to this the fact that few natural foods contain significant amounts of vitamin D, and a deficiency is a real possibility. Most plants are almost devoid of vitamin D, and few foods of animal origin contain much – fatty fish and cod liver oil are the best known. Even fresh milk does not naturally contain much vitamin D; the 400 International Units (IU) listed on each quart of milk are intentionally added to it.

You might ask, "why hasn't widespread vitamin D deficiency been evident before?" It has! Before vitamin D was added to milk (and now some breakfast cereals), rickets was prevalent in northern states where sunlight was minimal. But the idea that vitamin D deficiency is related to other diseases has blossomed only in the last 10 years or so. And it wasn't obvious at all that a vitamin might prevent an infectious disease. After all, that's the realm of antibiotics and antivirals, not vitamins. I don't want to overstate this situation. The evidence is only suggestive, but it is compelling.

It was recognized a century ago, before vitamin D was discovered, that children who had rickets also had more upper respiratory infections. Medical researchers now think these infections were related to the deficiency of vitamin D. Then, in one startling case several years ago, when the flu swept through a hospital, the patients of a physician who were being treated experimentally with vitamin D did not get the disease. Several new and intriguing studies continue to support the idea that the flu can at least be diminished with adequate intake of vitamin D.

Another reason for overlooking vitamin D's role in diseases besides rickets was that nutritionists thought it was very toxic at low levels. The requirement for vitamin D has been set at 400 IU/day for children and 200 IU/day for adults, and its toxicity started at 1,000-2,000 IU/day. At least that's what the textbooks say. But now after more research, it's to the contrary, and the toxic limit seems to be much higher (maybe 10,000 IU/day or more) and the daily need may be soon be set at 1,000 IU or more. These discoveries are so recent that newer numbers for toxicity and requirements have not been established, but they are being studied vigorously for revision. Some reputable medical researchers even suggest that very high levels of vitamin D be taken at the onset of the flu for three days to stop it. But we shall see. This is not a recommendation to do this. Because this is new evidence, one should be careful about taking supplements without discussing it first with a health provider.

With the prediction of widespread flu cases each winter, and the newer knowledge about vitamin D and disease, there are sure to be many observations about the flu and vitamin D as time goes on. Oh well, maybe all this news about vitamin D and the flu will turn out to be science fiction. But remember the stories about Buck Rogers a century or so ago? It was science fiction when he flew to the moon in a rocket. Now it's the truth!

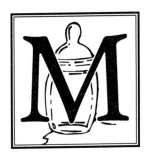

Melamine
A Tragic Food Story

The word melamine pops up in news articles now and then. You may have noticed it, but perhaps like most people, you probably didn't read the full story even though it mentioned something about babies dying in China. It seems relatively distant and unrelated to us until you know the whole story. And then it gets scary. Here's what's been happening.

In 2006, people in China illegally added melamine to pet foods in place of the protein from soybeans, wheat, and other ingredients. Melamine is high in nitrogen as is protein, and this was done to replace protein with the cheaper melamine. However, melamine is not a protein. It is a chemical used in the manufacture of plastics such as Formica and is not meant to be eaten. Although adequate nitrogen was present in the pet food, it came from melamine, a poison, and not the nutrient, protein – a very deceptive practice.

When cats and dogs consumed the melamine-adulterated pet food, many died. This started in China. But in this global economy, many pet food ingredients used in the U.S. come from China. During 2006-2007 there was a massive outbreak of kidney disease in cats and dogs in the United States. By mid-2007 over 17,000 cases of sick cats and dogs were reported with at least 4,500 deaths related to melamine. Did you know about this epidemic? The actual numbers were probably much larger.

The U.S. Food and Drug Administration (FDA) was not on the ball, and the related pet health problems went on and on. At first it was not known to be melamine. Several universities became involved and solved the mystery after much investigation and denial on part of the FDA. In 2007 it became obvious that people in China had been illegally adding melamine to pet food ingredients to boost the apparent protein content and make a big profit. On July 10, 2007, Zheng Xiaoyu, ex-head of the Chinese State Food and Drug Administration was executed for his part in this!

In 2007, cat and dog food from 89 and 102 companies, respectively, had been recalled! But where did that food go? It may have gotten into the U.S. human food supply. Exactly how is not known. But it seems certain that some melamine-contaminated pet food in the U.S. was not destroyed, instead it was sold as feed for pigs and chickens. Before it was discovered that this had been done the animals were sold for meat. Yes, you and I may have eaten some. This entire chain of events is described in the 2008 book, *Pet Food Politics*, by Marion Nestle, professor of nutrition, food studies and public health at New York University.

In spite of China's harsh action in 2007, the adulteration of Chinese food ingredients continued and in 2008 much of the infant milk formula in China was contaminated with melamine: 300,000 children got sick and some died. The chairwoman of China's largest dairy company was brought to trial for this.

There is now more control over melamine contamination, but it still shows up in small amounts in foods and dairy products around the world including the U.S. The escape clause by the U.S. government and food manufacturers is that low levels of melamine in foods (less than one part per million) are not harmful. But nobody has done that research. To quote from the 11/27/08 edition of the Washington Post, "Public health groups, consumer advocates, and members of Congress blasted the FDA yesterday for failing to act after discovering trace amounts of the industrial chemical melamine in baby formula in the United States." But there shouldn't be any at all!

Where are we now? Not in the best of shape! Problems still exist. Recently the Wall Street Journal (8/15/2010) reported that Dr. Margaret Hamburg, commissioner of the U.S. FDA said that the FDA does not have adequate resources to inspect the food supply from China for melamine, and the Chinese government is taking over collaborative responsibility for this work before foods leave China. Really! The assumption is that China has the situation under control. However, according to ABC News, and Reuters, Beijing (August 2010), many tons of melamine-contaminated milk are still found in China. Could this make its way into our foods?

I cannot put any humor into this article as I usually do. I just hope you educate yourself more on this matter, read the full stories that come out on melamine, and be careful choosing where your food comes from. This certainly champions the call for more local food production!

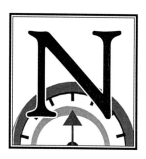

New Year's Resolutions
A Weighty Subject

The number one New Year's resolution is to lose weight. Many people fight this problem all year long. The lucky ones who don't have this problem can resolve to sleep more, see more movies, visit more friends, keep the house cleaner, or enjoy a variety of other cozy resolutions.

For the rest facing that painful weight loss, what diet will do the job? The answer is – any of them! But there is a qualifier: so long as you stick to the diet. I don't think a diet has been published that didn't work if you followed the directions, although they may not be the healthiest. I have in my office at least 100 different diet books. Some have familiar names like the *Atkin's diet*, but I also have *The Lazy Lady's Easy Diet* (sorry, I never saw one for the lazy man), *The Martinis and Whipped Cream Diet* (wow! what a way to do it), *The 21ˢᵗ Century Diet* (I guess it didn't work last century).

Studies published in the Journal of the American Medical Association compared four popular diets for a year with overweight women. Called the A to Z study, it looked at the following approaches: (1) the Atkin's diet – very low in carbohydrate but high in fat and protein with unlimited animal products; (2) the Zone diet – low in carbohydrate but with moderate and balanced amounts of fat and protein; (3) the LEARN diet – low in fat, high in carbohydrate, but it incorporates accepted principles of Lifestyle, Exercise, Attitudes, Relationships, and Nutrition; (4) the

Ornish diet – the standard for diets very low in fat, and very high in carbohydrate – almost the opposite of the Atkin's Diet. And the results? Numerically, the Atkin's diet won out; it produced the greatest weight loss, although the differences were small and not always statistically significant – almost a draw. Surprisingly, regarding health, the Atkin's Diet came out on top because it produced the best blood lipid profile – lower cholesterol, lower triglycerides, and better lipoproteins. Wow! What a surprise!

However, the main problem with diets is that when you "go off the diet" you go right back to old habits such as eating sweets, fats, refined foods, and such great breakfasts as two donuts and a whipped-top coffee, worth about 1,000 kilocalories. Most ex-dieters regain lost weight in a short period. The most important conclusion here is that people should not go on and off diets, but should modify their behavior so as not to gain the weight back in the first place. And this means controlling food intake, using will power, and exercising. Easy? No. But sorry, there isn't a magic pill yet! Do we have to list the rules? A glass of milk is better than a soft drink; a snack of bananas, apples, or berries is better than a bag of chips; candies, cakes, and white flour should not replace whole unrefined fiber-laden cereals and breads; ease up on fatty, fried foods, and so on. You know them, don't you?

While on the subject of behavior modification, keep in mind the importance of exercise: this can be more important than food choices. Many studies show that dieting or proper eating alone can not reduce weight or keep it under control – it must be linked with consistent exercise.

So is there anything New for this Year's resolutions? No! Choosing the right foods and coupling a balanced diet with regular exercise is nothing new. That was resolved years ago. This year let your New Year's Resolution become a healthy New Life Resolution instead. And the good news is that there's no need to wait for December 31 to resolve to do that. Happy New Life – today!

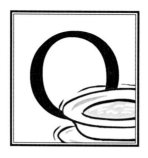

Mares Eat Oats
And Does Eat Oats
You Should Too!

O ats have long been considered one of the healthiest foods avail-able. As a result, the Food and Drug Administration (FDA) allows manufacturers of whole oat cereals such as Cheerios to put a label on the carton saying, in part, "may reduce the risk of heart disease." But this happened long after the popular song "Mairzy Doates" (written by Al Drake in 1943 for his daughter) told us that young horses and deer also eat lots of oats.

The FDA approved the "good for your heart" label because oats contain a unique kind of fiber. Oat grain is different from other plant grains such as wheat, corn, barley, etc., in that its fiber is mainly soft and soluble – like the pectins used to make jams and jellies. Most grains have insoluble, or tough, coarse fibers made largely of cellulose such as found in wheat bran. In their own way, these tough fibers are important to intestinal health because intestinal muscles have to work to process the fibers, and in doing so they are strengthened. To the contrary, an important function of soft, soluble fibers, found almost exclusively in fruits and vegetables, is to adsorb intestinal cholesterol and carry it out of the body. This supposedly helps prevent your blood cholesterol from rising and consequently prevents heart disease, although the evidence for dietary cholesterol causing heart disease has weakened substantially in the last few years. But this is why oats get this "good for your heart" label.

If you've followed nutritional news in the last few years you know that the indigestible part of plant food called fiber is so good for your health that it's almost considered an essential nutrient. Yes, this cardboard-like part of grains and cereals used to be considered a bothersome waste product, and we thought it just uselessly passed though our intestines and out the other end. Not anymore. Adequate dietary fiber may help prevent appendicitis, diverticulitis (infected pouches in the wall of the large intestine), polyps, gallstones, diabetes, and constipation, as well as heart disease.

Recently, the nutritional value of oats has taken on new significance. Scientists in the United States Department of Agriculture (USDA) discovered that oats contain a new family of antioxidants called avenanthramides (aka, Avns). Avns fight inflammation as do all antioxidants. Based on new scientific data, excessive, misplaced inflammation in your body is the main cause of many diseases. Inflammation is the response seen when you have an injury wherein irritation, swelling, redness, heat, and pain occur. That's fine. That's part of the healing process. But if this occurs when not needed, for example, in your arteries, soft organs, or other critical locations, it can lead to conditions such as hardening of the arteries and atherosclerosis. There is a strong body of evidence suggesting that inflammation may be the real cause of heart disease and that blood cholesterol is only a marker (and perhaps a poor one) for this.

At Tufts University, Dr. Mohsen Meydani reported that the antioxidant properties of Avns prevent blood cells from sticking to the lining of arteries. This gluing of cells to blood vessels is very likely the process that leads to blocking of the arteries in coronary heart disease. These researchers also suggest that Avns in oats relax you arteries. My gosh, isn't that what a day at the beach is supposed to do?

Cancer is another disease in which errant inflammation may play a role, and USDA researchers have evidence that oats may slow the growth of cancer cells in the colon. To add to the enthusiasm about oats, Time magazine recently published a lead story on aging. In it, 106-

year-old Leonard McCracken of Tavares, Florida is quoted as attributing his longevity to eating oats. Wow! Will eating oats slow our aging? I wonder if oat-eating mares and does live longer too?

A little caution though. There are estimated to be hundreds of antioxidants in various foods – most of them never studied. The Avns in oats could just be doing the same thing as antioxidants in other foods. We don't know. Please don't start dumping oats on all your meals. On the other hand, like mares and does, you might want to pay more attention to eating oats. Certainly, a whole grain cereal like oatmeal is a better choice than refined cereals that contain lots of sugar! So pay attention when you hear the old song "Mairzy Doats and Dozy Doats," but for heaven's sake don't be like little lambs and kids and start eating ivy.

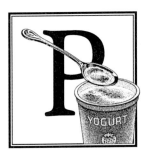

Pro-Biotics
What Are They For?

If the word antibiotic means "against life," and antibiotics kill harmful organisms, then the word probiotic must mean "for life" and probiotics keep beneficial organisms alive. Correct? Well, in a way that's true. The word probiotic actually refers to the bacteria themselves, the beneficial ones that are helpful and not harmful, and when ingested improve your health. For example, the harmful bacteria, *Staphylococcus*, can cause "staph" infections in the skin and are killed by antibiotics such as penicillin. But helpful bacteria, such as *Lactobacillus* found in dairy products, can reduce intestinal infections and keep our body's cells from being destroyed.

Probiotics (friendly bacteria) are most often found in foods. The best example is the bacteria in yogurt. Yogurt is almost identical to milk except that certain bacteria have been allowed to grow in it during fermentation. The bacteria convert the milk into a semisolid with a characteristic acidic taste that we call yogurt. If the bacteria are friendly or health promoting then consuming foods such as yogurt should improve health.

There are two main types of bacteria found in common supermarket yogurt: *Lactobacillus bulgaricus* and *Streptococcus thermophilus*. Others that are stronger probiotics such as *Lactobacillus acidophilus* are frequently added. One thing bacteria from yogurt can do is colonize in the intestine and replace harmful bacteria that may be there. Yogurt is frequently used in medicine and especially pediatrics for the treatment of intestinal problems. The probiotics in yogurt activate the immune system and are helpful in preventing conditions such as lactose intolerance, irritable bowel syndrome, indigestion, diarrhea, and even colic in babies. They also help reestablish the community of beneficial bacteria in the intestine after antibiotics have been used.

But this story becomes most interesting when we realize that there may be hundreds of different types of bacteria that have health promoting properties. A yogurt-related dairy product called Kefir, which can be purchased locally, contains 10 or more different probiotic bacteria.

There are many yogurts produced around the world. They are made from different combinations of good bacteria and from different types of milk (cow, mare, goat, and sheep). Among them are Kumis from Russia and Mongolia, Yakult from Japan, Boruga from the Dominican Republic, and Kushuk from Iraq.

The story of yogurt and probiotics started about 1900 with the Nobel Prize-winning Russian scientist, Elie Metchnikoff. He observed that people living in Bulgaria who ate yogurt seemed to live longer. Metchnikoff believed this was due to the bacteria in yogurt and was among the first to discover that bacteria were responsible for the fermentation of milk to yogurt. Based on this work, one of the bacteria found in yogurt was named *Lactobacillus bulgaricus* (because it was first found in Bulgaria). You will find this listed on most yogurt labels. Although the effect of yogurt on longevity turned out not to be true, Metchnikoff's writings initiated interest in the role of yogurt bacteria in health.

The field of probiotics is one of the hottest in food science. You will be seeing more ads stating that these or those probiotic bacteria have special health-promoting properties. And apart from finding them in yogurts, you will find them being added to other foods such as snacks, health bars, cereals, cheese, baby formulas, etc. Probiotics are now used widely in animal feeds, including those for horses and chickens. They are even sold in capsules.

The advice here is not to believe all the puffery you may read about probiotics until its proven true through adequate testing in humans. But for now, the more natural sources and types of beneficial bacteria in a food, the better. Read the label. Regardless, no matter in what form you consume probiotics, they definitely favor your well-being.

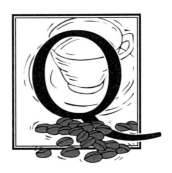

Quit Drinking Coffee?
Maybe, But Maybe Not!

O f all the foods I've lectured about, coffee is one of the most frustrating. Good and bad information about coffee seems to change each year. One year it causes heart disease and the next year it prevents it. One year it causes miscarriages and the next year it prevents Parkinson's disease. What is one to do? Should we quit drinking coffee or drink more of it? I don't have an exact answer, but here is the current situation.

First of all, one difficulty in discussing coffee is that we equate it almost directly with caffeine, as if any problem or benefit is due to that. In reality, coffee contains over 1,000 different substances, and caffeine, although the most notable, is only one of them. About two percent of coffee is made up of caffeine; other substances make up the rest.

On the positive side, coffee contains chemicals such as chlorogenic acid and caffeic acid that are strong antioxidants. We know that antioxidants are essential to health and that they may prevent heart disease, aging, and cancer. A recent study from Finland and Sweden suggested that antioxidants in coffee might explain why coffee drinkers seem to have less Alzheimer's disease.

There is also reasonable evidence that coffee drinkers develop less Parkinson's disease. And the risk of gallstones may be less as well. Furthermore, as any coffee drinker knows, energy, mental performance, and especially moods are elevated throughout the day by that morning cup of coffee. Even athletes have found that coffee improves their physical performance. Most, but not necessarily all of these effects can be attributed to caffeine.

On the negative side, a couple of lipids in coffee, strangely called cafestol and kahweol, have been shown to elevate blood cholesterol. According to this information, if you have blood cholesterol problems, coffee is bad for you. But, population studies with large groups of people have not detected any increased heart disease among coffee drinkers. One recent study even suggested that people who have heart attacks are better off if they have been drinking coffee.

Only about 20 of those 1,000 substances in coffee have ever been studied in detail and this has been done only in research animals. In these cases, increases in cancer rates have been observed. However, studies with humans have shown no effect of coffee intake on longevity and health. Therefore, what happens in an experimental rat or pig may be quite different from what happens to you.

Unfortunately, some people cannot tolerate caffeine and must either use decaffeinated coffee or avoid it altogether. Caffeinated coffee can exacerbate problems of atrial fibrillation, which causes the upper heart chambers to beat excessively at hundreds of beats per minute. This can lead to serious consequences such as blood clots. Almost as important, coffee may increase miscarriages, decrease fertility, and lower birth weights of babies. These effects usually are blamed on caffeine, but require the consumption of several cups of coffee per day. Intake of regular coffee also causes insomnia, and there is concern that many people with sleep problems are simply over consuming coffee.

Regularly drinking caffeinated coffee can be addictive, and stopping "cold turkey" can cause tiredness, headaches, nausea, muscle aches, and even poor concentration for two weeks or more. Many psychiatrists don't like the word "addictive" used in this context because caffeine certainly is not in the same category as cocaine.

So, should you or shouldn't you drink coffee? Pregnant women should limit consumption. People with heart beat irregularities, sleep, mood, or behavioral problems, should consider limiting coffee consumption also because it could play a role in the problem.

On balance, drinking coffee holds benefits for many people too, even if it is just that boost in the morning.

Socially, a cup of coffee helps smooth our daily interactions with others. And, oh yes! Just this week, it was reported that something in coffee prevents bad breath. So drinking coffee may be more important to our social life than we ever knew!

Note to parents and teenagers about caffeine – Just released from Drexel University in the journal, *Pediatrics*. Thirty percent of teenagers fall asleep during school, and caffeine consumption the preceding night was 76 percent higher among those students.

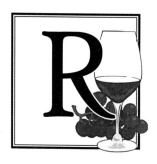

Resveratrol
Stayin' Alive, Stayin' Alive

F ew people have heard of this new nutritional buzzword, resveratrol, but many have heard and danced to the Bee Gees famous disco song "Stayin' Alive." So what do the two have in common? They both address one of our greatest desires – to stay alive as long as possible, at least as long as we are healthy.

Resveratrol is a chemical substance found in many foods such as cranberries, peanuts, and dark fruits, and it is increasingly promoted as a new "magic bullet" to lengthen your life span. The original impetus to study this strange chemical came from a long-standing nutritional controversy called the "French Paradox." The French Paradox addresses the nutritional fact that people in France have less heart disease and they live longer than we do, in spite of the fact that the French eat a lot more rich, creamy, and buttery foods. If you follow French cooking at all you know they use fatty, high-energy ingredients in many recipes.

In looking for an answer to the French Paradox, one possibility that quickly came to mind was that the French drink a lot of red wine. And yes, red wine contains a fair amount of resveratrol – and resveratrol was found to increase the lifespan of yeast. Could sumptuous consumption of red wine be the answer? So, from this very positive correlation between the French drinking red wine, its resveratrol content and a longer life in yeast, it looked like everyone should mimic the French and drink lots of red wine to live longer – let's have a glass at breakfast, lunch, and dinner! Actually, resveratrol was discovered in the 1940s, long before the French Paradox surfaced. It's an antioxidant, but it also seems to act as an antibiotic in plants to help them fight infections. Thankfully, grapes themselves contain resveratrol, so you don't have to live with a life-long alcoholic buzz on in order to get resveratrol. A glass of grape juice should do just fine.

As nice and logical as this story sounded, serious questions arose. First, most of the research showing that resveratrol improves health and increases longevity has been done in lower animals, from worms to mice. Well, that's nice for mice, but what about men? No long-term studies have been done in humans, neither in men nor women. Secondly, it would take the equivalent of several hundred glasses of red wine (or grape juice) per day to supply the high amount of resveratrol that seemed to work in these animals. So, poof, there goes the French Paradox theory. And I've never seen any of my healthy French friends drink that much!

Resveratrol has been extracted from plants and can be purchased in pill form in large amounts. It's sold to improve your health and extend your lifespan. But what about its safety? A couple of small studies in people suggest that it's safe; however, there are no data about its long-term effects. I'm reminded of the widespread use many years ago of the comfrey plant. Its leaves and roots were thought to be very healthful as components of salads and teas, and you could easily grow it in your garden. Many people used it. It was a natural herbal plant, so of course it was considered safe. Then a Japanese study found that comfrey contains toxins (one called symphytine), which cause liver cancer. Well, resveratrol may not be symphytine, but we don't know much about its effects in humans. Maybe we should just stick with a little wine or grape juice now and then and not be tempted by "magic bullets." After all, bullets can do harm.

So, we have to make good decisions about stayin' alive. Maybe it would be better to dance to the Bee Gees' disco music than take a resveratrol pill. Dancing the disco like John Travolta in the movie *Saturday Night Fever* would probably extend our lifespan much longer than any magic bullet could. Try that!

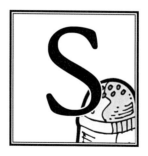

Salt
Have You Stopped Shaking Yet?

I don't mean "Have you stopped using the salt shaker?" but I do mean, "Have you stopped shaking your head?" about the controversy surrounding table salt? One day nutritionists state that excessive salt causes high blood pressure, and the next day they report that it's harmless. My head is still shaking about this. What is going on?

Certainly, common table salt or sodium chloride, NaCl, is an essential mineral and without it you die. But in terms of excess, sodium is the problem. Too much sodium can increase blood pressure and cause heart disease and stroke. But the whole story is long and very complex, so let's focus on why we want so much salt and what to do to stay healthy.

The story starts with the little-appreciated fact that natural fruits and vegetables are almost devoid of sodium, and natural meats have only a little more. Most salt is obtained from seawater by evaporation or mined from salt mountains and underground briny springs. Until recently, unless you lived near one of these sources, your diet was probably deficient in sodium. We thus evolved with a built-in, biological, compulsive drive to seek sodium in order to survive, much like the drive to seek water. But with the advent of cheap transportation many years ago, salt was easily shipped around the world and became readily available and cheap. Thus, our compulsion to find salt in order to survive became a lust for too much salt.

Whether or not you are harmed by excess salt intake is partially genetically determined. Of the 30-40 percent of adults in the U.S. estimated to have high blood pressure, as many as 75 percent of them are genetically sensitive to table salt (it varies with age, ethnicity, obesity, and other factors). If high-blood pressure runs in your family, your risk is increased. To the contrary, many people are also genetically resistant to the bad effects of excessive sodium, and this creates the controversy in scientific studies. But even if high blood pressure isn't present in your family, there is no way currently to determine if excess sodium can harm you. It's best to be careful.

To add to the confusion, the easiest solution should be to reduce dietary sodium – but that's not quite true. Although it certainly helps, increasing your intake of the mineral potassium may be as important. Sodium and potassium work together in the body to maintain optimal health. Normally, you should have about three times as much potassium in your food as sodium, or a 3:1 ratio. But nowadays with salt readily available, and considering our built-in drive to get it, this ratio is almost reversed to 1:2. This is not consistent with good health. It's easy to increase potassium intake. Those very fruits and vegetables so low in sodium are also high in potassium, so just consume several servings a day. I think a banana named Chiquita proclaimed that many years ago.

The saltshaker accounts for only a small part of excessive sodium intake – maybe 15 percent on average. Salt added to processed foods is a major culprit. So it's important to read labels and choose low-salt foods. For example, a single cup of regular tomato sauce contains 1,440 mg. of sodium or almost 100 percent your recommended intake of 1,500 mg., while the one labeled "no salt added" has only 80 mg. or 6.6 percent of your needs. A single 120 kilocalorie serving of "vegetarian lentil stew" contains 450 mg. or 30 percent of the recommended intake for sodium. That's a lot! Food manufacturers are slowly trying to change this, but don't be too hard on them, especially bakers. Without some salt many recipes such as breads and cakes simply won't work.

So if you meet me walking down the street and I don't say hello, I'm probably still shaking my head thinking about all the confusing information I processed as I wrote this story. But please, do stop and shake my hand!

ADDENDUM

Soybeans ~ Should You Or Shouldn't You?

A reader asked me to comment on the safety of eating soybeans. Soybeans are an excellent source of protein, energy, vitamins, and minerals, but they also contain other chemicals that can be harmful. Soybeans must be heated for humans and other animals in order to destroy at least two factors that interfere with digestion and thyroid function. When soymilk is manufactured, the beans are boiled. Beyond this, soy products contain hormones known as phytoestrogens or flavonoids, which don't seem to be destroyed by heating. It is controversial whether these phytoestrogens are beneficial or harmful to humans. They have been shown to both prevent and promote breast cancer, and nutrition writers really take sides on the soy issue. I found one well-known nutrition group that knocked soybeans saying they interfered with digestion – but that is true only if they are eaten raw, which they are not. Another group strongly promoted soybeans, but they were selling books that knocked milk. Some bias, huh? By the way, if soybeans are properly heated, the protein is not destroyed as some claim. I have worked for years with heated soybeans as the main protein source in diets for chickens and pigs, and they do just fine. On the other hand, children and babies can be very sensitive to the phytoestrogens, and soy should be used cautiously at these ages, usually where milk allergies or lactose intolerance are problems. As indicated in an excellent article the reader sent in, there may be important individual variations, good and bad, between people and their response to soybeans that we cannot measure and about which we are still uncertain. The best current advice is to use soybean products in moderation as part of a balanced diet, limit use with babies and young children, and keep your eyes open for new scientific developments.

Trans Fats
A Good Story With Bad, Bad Characters

Almost everybody has heard the story of trans fats. You've correctly been told to look at labels and avoid foods that contain them. Over the last 40-50 years these bad characters were likely a major factor in causing heart disease. This seems so certain that cities such as New York have banned trans fats in foods sold there. This story is filled with scheming, political intrigue, and death. Wow! Where did this tragic drama come from?

What we call fats, such as vegetable oils, butter, margarine, beef and pork fat, etc. are really molecules made primarily of fatty acids. What's important to the plot of this story is that different types of fatty acids can have both good and bad effects on your health. Some of the good ones are monounsaturated, polyunsaturated and omega-3 fatty acids. But among the bad fatty acids are those called trans; they are bad enough that if you eat them they can cause heart disease.

Until recently, we didn't hear much about trans fats. Unlike all the other fats mentioned above, they've been kept in the dark, out of view, because most trans fatty acids are not natural; they are artificial, synthetic fats! Although a few are found in small amounts naturally, the trans fatty acids we encounter in most foods are "man-made" by chemists. They only occur when natural fats such as corn and soybean oils are heated excessively and treated with hydrogen. This is done to make liquid oils more solid so that they resemble butter and lard. Thus, oleomargarine (or simply margarine) was born near the beginning of the last century to compete with butter.

Artificial trans fatty acids do not occur in nature and our bodies are not familiar with them. Thus, when we eat them and they get into our tissues, they raise havoc with the structure of muscle cells and cause heart disease. There is also some evidence they cause cancer.

Although margarine was available early in the last century, it was not used much until after World War II because it was taxed to make it more expensive than butter. In the 1950s President Truman removed this tax and margarine became cheap and widely used. Originally, margarine was taxed because Vermont's then-Governor George Aiken promoted this to support the dairy industry and protect the sale of butter.

In the late 1960s, researchers at the University of Illinois first showed that artificial trans fats can lead to heart disease in pigs, but such evidence was kept quiet until the 1990s and people continued eating margarines with the bad trans fatty acids in them. I taught this information throughout my 40 years as a professor, and I regret that I didn't publish this knowledge more widely.

Fortunately, in the last 15-20 years, people have been made aware to avoid trans fatty acids, but they still exist widely in foods, especially cookies, snacks, popcorn, and crackers that use a semisolid fat.

Many foods are listed as having zero trans fats in them and in many cases, this is a lie. Zero is not really zero for government-regulated food labeling. Food manufacturers can list zero trans fats if there is less than ½ gram per serving. What you must do is look at the label to see if partially-hydrogenated vegetable oils are being used; if so, then there are trans fats in the food, regardless of the label. Other fats such as saturated or coconut fats do not supply "artificial trans fats." The Institute of Medicine recommends that intake of trans fatty acids be kept to a minimum.

I have emphasized *artificial* trans fats which are produced during processing. In natural fats such as milk or beef fat there are small amounts of natural trans fatty acids – these are good for you health, and they can actually help prevent heart disease! One is known as conjugated linoleic acid (CLA). So there are a few good trans fat characters in our story.

The trans fatty acid story does not have a simple plot, and the whole tale is complicated by mystery, intrigue, and lies. Be a sleuth and keep your eyes on food labels: beware of those bad partially hydrogenated characters lurking in the market. Be as afraid as if this story began with "On a dark and stormy night."

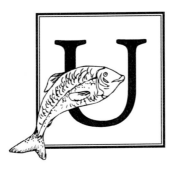

Unsaturated Fats
Omega-3s Are Tops

By now almost everybody has heard about omega-3 fatty acids, especially in relation to eating fish. But is this really an important subject? Or is it a lot of hype like low fat and low carbohydrate diets, egg cholesterol, or other nutritional topics touting benefits or harm that seem to wax and wane and change yearly? In this case, the answer is that this is one of the most important subjects to everyone's health, and it does deserve a lot of attention.

Omega-3 fatty acids are very long and highly unsaturated. They differ structurally from the more common fatty acids we find in everyday foods. The omega-3 tells us they have a double bond in their structure three spaces from the end (omega in Greek means end or last).

More important is that omega-3 fatty acids are found in very few foods, and they are limited to fish oils, flaxseed, and a few other plants. The other fats and oils that are commonly found in most vegetable oils, meats, and foods contain mainly omega-6 and omega-9 fatty acids. Now, couple this with today's understanding that the omega-3s are essential to health, that they must be supplied by foods and are not manufactured in our bodies, and this becomes a critical issue. People who eat the typical U.S. diet high in meats and vegetable oils, and lacking fish, are most likely deficient in omega-3 fatty acids. Yes, if that's your situation, you may be living every day with a nutritional deficiency.

There are two principle omega-3 fatty acids, both found exclusively in fish oil: docosahexaenoic acid (DHA), and eicosapentaenoic acid (EPA). The importance of these is that DHA is a structural component of nervous tissue and other cells in the body, and EPA is especially needed to fight inflammation. A lot has been written about omega-3s preventing heart disease and that is true. A study from Tufts University showed that omega 3 fatty acids "reduce the rates of all-cause mortality, cardiac and sudden death, and possibly stroke." Omega-3s also reduce blood cholesterol and control heart fibrillations, and have been reported to prevent prostate and breast cancer.

Less well known is the important role omega-3s play in the function of the nervous system. Evidence is accumulating rapidly that intake of sufficient quantities of omega-3s helps reduce many nervous disorders such as depression, dementia, schizophrenia, Alzheimer's disease, attention deficit disorder, bipolar disorder, and violent behavior in prison inmates. Omega-3s also play an important role in memory, and several studies have associated adequate omega-3 intake with increased learning by schoolchildren. Some synthetic baby formulas now include omega-3s because they are important for the baby's brain and eye development, and they reduce behavioral problems. So fish and its oils really are brain foods.

Omega-3s found in some plants such as flax seed, walnuts, purslane, and grasses are not the same as those in fish oil. Plants contain the omega-3 called alpha linolenic acid (ALA). This molecule is smaller than the fish oil omega-3s, and to be beneficial ALA must first be converted in the body into DHA and EPA, the forms found in fish. One limitation is that this conversion is very inefficient, about 10 percent or so, and one would have to eat many plants to get enough. But because fish get their omega-3s from algae and other phytoplankton, one could also consume the algae directly and such supplements are available on the market.

The usual recommendation for fish omega-3s is 0.5-1 grams per day (more in some disease situations). This can be obtained by eating two-four servings of certain cold-water ocean fish per week or by capsules of fish oil. Crustaceans such as lobster and crabs contain less than fish. And while some freshwater fish like trout contain omega-3s, tilapia has almost none.

So you really should pay attention to this nutritional news: omega-3 fatty acids are really essential for good mental health – remember that!

Omega-3 Fatty Acid Content of Some Foods grams/100 grams

Salmon	1.4
Lobster	0.2
Sardines	1.7
Crab	0.4
Mackerel	2.2
Shrimp	0.5
Anchovies	1.4
Oyster	0.6
Tuna	1.6
Flax seed	20.0*
Cod	0.3
Purslane	0.4*
Flounder	0.2
Canola oil	10.0*
Perch	0.4
Wheat germ oil	7.0*
Trout, lake	1.6
Walnuts	6.0*

* As ALA

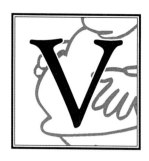

Visceral Fat
Oh No… Not Another Bad Fat!

You've read the story about fats over and over. Many advise that omega-3 fats from fish are good for your health and trans fats in margarine are bad. Polyunsaturated vegetable oils are good for your heart and saturated animal fats are bad. Some of this advise is questionable, but haven't we heard enough already? Well, no! This isn't where the story of fats ends. There is also something called visceral fat, and too much of it is very bad. So let's look at this new chapter in the good/bad story about fats. Did you ever wonder why excess body fat or obesity causes a host of diseases such as diabetes, heart disease, high blood pressure, asthma, and kills people? Turn the pages.

Visceral fat is not fat that you eat, it's fat that you make yourself. You may not be a butcher or baker, but you are a visceral fat maker. Visceral fat is the adipose tissue that surrounds the organs in your abdomen, and it has special properties different from that of body fat found elsewhere. It secretes substances that in small amounts are essential to survival, but in larger amounts can ruin your health.

Most of the time we think of body fat as simply a place where excess energy or calories are stored; kind of an inert place like a dish of butter or a packet of olive oil that is hanging around just waiting to be used up. That's true for subcutaneous fat located just under your skin. It stays there until you run out of food, and then it's used up to supply missing energy you need.

But, visceral fat is quite the opposite. Although it also stores calories, it is a thriving, metabolically active, churning chemical factory, and it produces many different substances that get into your blood and circulate throughout the body. Most notably, visceral fat produces chemicals involved with inflammation. Inflammation is one of the newer buzzwords that's most often associated with a lot of health problems. But in reality inflammation in small amounts is an essential process required for survival. This is what occurs when your body is injured either externally or internally. You see the inflammatory process when a wound becomes red, inflamed, hot, and sore. This occurs because many different kinds of molecules and cells race to the injury site to start the healing process. That's good. Without this, an injury would never heal.

The problem arises when you have too much visceral fat, which like other fat in your body, increases in body mass if you overeat. What you eat does not matter here – sugar, fat, protein – it's the amount that's important because all excess is converted to fat.

Many of the potentially harmful chemicals produced by visceral fat are known. They go under such complicated names as cytokines, leukotrienes, tumor necrosis factor, interleukins, C-reactive protein, and other names best left to the biochemists to worry about. In small amounts they help cure injuries, but in large amounts they do excessive damage – they act as if the whole body has been injured.

The main problem here is central obesity or belly fat. Fat around the hips and buttocks is not such a severe health problem because it is less metabolically active than visceral fat and behaves more like subcutaneous fat. Curiously, hip fat occurs mainly due to an increase in numbers of fat cells whereas visceral fat is more related to an increase in fat cell size. Yes, even fat cells have their own personalities.

You are well aware of the plot to this story – too much visceral fat is dangerous. Have you been anticipating the conclusion? You know what it is, don't you? Does it help if we hint that visceral fat is especially responsive to exercise? We don't have to read further as the last few lines of the story are obvious. So close the book on good fats/bad fats and reach your own conclusion as to what should be written in the final sentence... you knew this all along.

V | ADDENDUM
Vegan Food Patterns

A reader asked me to discuss the vegetarian eating pattern known as the vegan diet. Although I'm not a vegetarian I'll try to make this valuable and give you your money's worth.

Vegans (VEE-guns) follow a diet pattern totally devoid of animal products. Some vegetarians include eggs and dairy, and even a little fish or chicken, but the true vegetarian or vegan eliminates all of these – no animal products, period! But rather than calling it a vegan diet, let's refer to it as a vegan food pattern. Diet sounds too severe, and makes one think weight loss is the primary objective.

People follow a vegan food pattern for several reasons: religious, environmental, animal welfare and personal health. The first three are absolutely valid reasons, but what about the last one, health? Is a vegan food pattern good or bad? It can be both. In its generic sense, a vegan food pattern includes any combination of plant products. It could consist of only white bread, butter substitute, and soybeans or nuts. That certainly supplies carbohydrate, fat, and protein, but obviously, it's not very balanced.

Most vegans start out intending to follow a balanced diet to improve their health, but frequently fall short. The exclusion of nutrient laden meat, eggs, and dairy products can lead to deficiencies. A vegan food pattern can be deficient in vitamin B-12, iron, calcium, zinc, vitamin D, omega-3 fatty acids, and balanced amino acids. As examples, a recent study showed that 80 percent of some vegans in India are deficient in vitamin B-12; this is dangerous and can cause irreversible nerve damage. Or, vegan children of vegan parents, who do not understand good nutrition, are known to do poorly in school. This is not necessarily a harsh criticism of the vegan food pattern but leads to the one important qualification for being a vegan – one must also be a pretty good nutritionist! Vegans must learn how to balance plant foods and educate themselves as to food sources of nutrients. Nutrition education? That's not such a bad idea for everyone. When this is done the vegan food pattern has a lot of pluses.

Proper vegan food patterns are known to lower blood pressure, and lessen the risk of developing heart disease, obesity, diabetes, cancer, intestinal problems, and many other current health problems. On that basis, the vegan food pattern is highly recommended. One reservation, however, is that comparisons of vegans are usually made to the general population in which highly imbalanced, high energy, low fiber diets are currently eaten. It's my opinion that any well balanced, unrefined diet that is faithfully adhered to, that is not excessive in calories, and that includes a lifestyle of physical activity along with no smoking or drugs, will produce similar results. I can't go into the concept of a balanced diet here. But you know pretty well what this means, don't you? It's not refined fast foods every day.

Most of the problematic nutrients in a vegan food pattern can be obtained by paying particular attention to using unrefined foods, a wide array of beans, seeds, nuts and super vegetables such as broccoli, although supplements of vitamin D (in the winter), and vitamin B-12 are frequently used. Good food choices nearly correct any possible deficits. Excellent vegan meal patterns examples are available online and in books.

At some meals I'm a vegan. A big green, red and purple salad with a side bowl of squash, along with grapes, cherries, and nuts is a favorite of mine. And of course being from Boston, beans light up my life.

So if a vegan food pattern is what makes you feel healthy and content, and you have learned some important nutritional principles, more power to you. But, other well-balanced food patterns that include eggs, milk, cheese, chicken, fish, or meat will produce similar results.

I hope this discussion was valuable to you, and you didn't mind me putting in my two cents worth. Next time, I may just ask you for a penny for my thoughts.

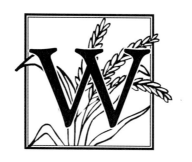

Wheat Is Fine
If Not Refined

Have you heard the news about white bread? The largest bakeries in the U.S. – the ones in California that make Wonder bread – are closing. Wow! There goes an icon. This in part signals the continuing consumer shift from soft, white breads made of highly refined, processed wheat flour to breads made of whole, unrefined grains. More and more people are getting and heeding the word that eating unrefined grain products is better for your health.

People make jokes about the consistency and lack of taste in loaves of refined white bread and yet it still shows up frequently in shopping carts. There once was a good reason for this. Whole grains have a fairly long shelf life, but once ground, they go rancid more quickly because the unsaturated oils in the grains oxidize when exposed to air. They don't pass the sniff test and smell rancid after an extended storage period. Consequently, grains were refined to remove the germ, where most of the oil resides, along with the bran. The remaining starchy part lasted much longer without going rancid and worked great in commercial breads. And people got used to eating them. But along the way something important was lost because most of the vitamins and minerals were removed from the whole grains and few remained in the starchy flour. Fortunately, nowadays, there are better storage and packaging methods, quicker transport, local production, and in non-organic breads, antioxidants and preservatives may be added. We can now return to eating whole grain products. You also have the added benefit of better flavor. There is no comparison between the nut-like flavor of whole wheat breads and the blandness of breads made with refined flour.

Removing the germ and bran from grains removes most of the 50 or so nutrients found in them. This was recognized as a problem in the U.S. in the 1940s because nutritional deficiencies of thiamin (vitamin B_1), riboflavin (vitamin B_2), and niacin (vitamin B_3) started showing up. These deficiencies had existed long before this, but in the years between 1912 and the 1940s, discoveries of the vitamins were taking place. Laws were then passed that these three vitamins had to be added back to white refined flour. But what about the rest of the nutrients? They were in the germ and bran, which were fed to pigs, and guess who was healthier – humans or pigs?

Take magnesium as one example. It is needed for the health of muscle, bones, and the nervous system. In refined wheat, 80 percent or so of the magnesium is removed and it's not added back. Low intake of magnesium is definitely associated with heart disease. Or look at vitamin B_6, known as pyridoxine. Most is lost during refining. It is not replaced because supposedly, stark deficiencies of it are not seen. However, borderline deficiencies of pyridoxine are known to exist and symptoms may be slight complaints of irritability and fatigue. Sound familiar?

Refined wheat is not the only culprit. In the early part of the last century, heavy consumption of corn grits, which is the starchy remnant of highly-refined corn grain, led to a deficiency of the B-vitamin, niacin and the worst nutritional epidemic in the U.S. This caused a disease called pellagra, with severe and dreadful symptoms of diarrhea, dermatitis, and dementia (resembling schizophrenia). Hundreds of thousands of people, mainly in southern states, got pellagra and many died before it was mandated that niacin be added back to refined grains.

We can't discuss every nutrient lost when grains like wheat are refined and stripped of the germ and bran, but this list would also include zinc, manganese, copper, selenium, chromium, vitamin E, pantothenic acid, choline, and others. Additionally, you won't get all the fiber and the many antioxidants supplied by whole grains. So the next time you buy breakfast cereal, pizza, bread, pasta, or rice be sure to grab the unrefined type. Your meal will be healthier and tastier.

Lyn Carew's Favorite Whole Wheat Bread

6-8 cups unsifted, stone ground whole wheat flour

3 tablespoons wheat germ

2 teaspoons salt

2 tablespoons active dry yeast

1½ cups cold water

1½ cups milk, scalded slightly

1/3 cup molasses

1/3 cup honey

1/3 cup canola oil *(olive and corn oils work)* or melted margarine *(modern type with no trans fatty acids)*

Proof yeast in large mixing bowl in a little warm water. Combine about 5 cups of flour with the wheat germ, salt, and yeast in mixing bowl.

Separately, combine and mix cold water, scalded milk, molasses, and honey. Gradually add the cooled liquid to dry ingredients and beat with electric mixer for several minutes at medium speed, scraping bowl occasionally. Add oil (now or earlier), and mix in enough additional flour to make the dough stiff enough to leave sides of bowl. Turn out onto lightly floured board, add additional flour as necessary, and knead until smooth and elastic, leaving the dough very slightly moist. Place in a lightly greased bowl, turning to grease the top. Cover with a towel, let rise in warm place until doubled in bulk (2-4 hrs.). Knead again, then shape dough into loaves to fit into greased pans filling them 1/3 - 1/2 full. Cover and let rise. Preheat oven to 350°. Bake for 30-45 minutes depending on size of loaf. When done place warm loaves on a raised rack and cover loosely with tin foil. Crust on loaves should be light brown. Makes 2-4 loaves. The cook can sample loaves just out of the oven.

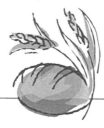

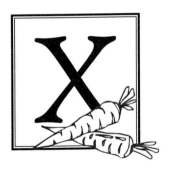

eXamine Vitamin A
It Can Be Toxic

If a vitamin is good for you, will a lot of it be even better? No! In most cases, that idea is wrong with nutrients! And high doses of vitamin A are a current worry among nutritionists. In earlier times, we did not think that vitamin A in excess, up to five times or more the daily requirement, was a problem. But recent results have shown that even small excesses can lead to a variety of health problems including hip and bone fractures, especially in women, and even birth defects if taken during pregnancy. In excess, vitamin A may be among the most toxic of the vitamins and the range between that which you require and a harmful level is narrow, sometimes only three to four times as much. So look at your vitamin supplements to see how much vitamin A you take each day. Your total daily need is 3,000-5,000 international units – the units usually found on food and pill labels – or 900-1,500 micrograms. The pure form of vitamin A is of most concern, and not the vitamin A source found in plants, meats, and eggs.

We all know that carrots and vitamin A are essential for good eyesight – that's taught in most schools. And it is a fact that deficient levels of vitamin A can lead to "night blindness" whereby we cannot adapt readily to seeing in dim light such as when entering a movie theater or other dark room in the middle of the day. Normally it takes a couple of minutes to adapt to the dim light and recognize that there are actually seats and people in the theater. With a vitamin A deficiency, this adaptation can take many more minutes.

Vitamin A is also needed for good skin health. As a result, some women erroneously take high doses of vitamin A to preserve beauty, and this has been promoted by the popular press. Such high intakes can be in the range of 25,000-50,000 international units (IU) per day, which is much higher than the established requirement of 3,000-5,000 IU/day. The culprit here is the form of vitamin A in pills and supplements. In vegetables like carrots and spinach, vitamin A is supplied in a form called beta-carotene, a yellow-orange pigment that is later converted to vitamin A in your body. Beta-carotene belongs to a whole group of nutrients called carotenoids – all plant pigments. However, in pills and other supplements it is frequently the vitamin A molecule itself, not carotene, which is supplied. Beta-carotene from foods, even in much higher amounts than the daily requirement, is rarely a problem because it must be processed into vitamin A. In fact, high intakes of foods containing beta-carotene are consistent with improved health. Of great importance is that beta-carotene and the vegetables that contain it also help prevent cancer. Yes, vitamin A itself is found in fatty animal products such as egg yolk and butter, but usually in small amounts.

So the lesson here is to get lots of vitamin A via the beta-carotene in vegetables, but be wary of vitamin A supplied directly in large amounts in supplements and pills. Green and yellow vegetables are your best source of beta-carotene, so load up on them. This is why nutritionists suggest five servings of vegetables a day. Examine your vitamin A intake so that you can see what's going on.

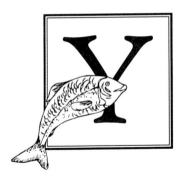

Yes Or No!
Fish Versus Mercury

I love seafood, but fish eaters are in a quandary these days. We are told to eat fish two-three times a week to get those omega-3 fatty acids that keep us healthy. But then we are told to be wary of mercury in fish. Mercury is certainly a dangerous chemical, and eating fish is the main route it takes into our diets. Shouldn't that keep us from eating fish? It sounds scary…what are we to do? Well, it hasn't been popularized much, but a mineral called selenium can save the day.

But first, what are these omega-3 fatty acids in fish? Fatty acids are the major components of fats in foods. That's what corn oil, soybean oil, butter fat, olive oil, margarine, and all the other fats you can think of are made of, including the fat or oil in fish. But fish contain very unique fatty acids called omega-3 fatty acids that go by the initials EPA and DHA. They are not supplied by other foods so we must eat fish to get them. Some fatty acids in foods such as flaxseed can be converted to EPA and DHA but this is very inefficient. Considerable research shows that EPA and DHA may help prevent heart disease and cancer, and almost certainly improves brain development and function, especially in babies. The latter point is so critical that many infant formulas are now supplemented with at least one of these omega-3s.

So how can we worry less? A most intriguing fact is that the mineral selenium, which is abundant in fish, is a strong antagonist of mercury.

Selenium is one of the 20 essential minerals we must get in our food to stay alive – it's a nutrient. The selenium in fish grabs the mercury, binds strongly to it, and inactivates it permanently. You can think of selenium as a magnet that attracts mercury. Most fish contain much more selenium than mercury so selenium wins out in this battle. Scientists at the University of North Dakota reported that tuna and flounder contain about 25 times as much selenium as mercury (although one study placed albacore tuna at 3:1 but another at 15:1) and salmon has 10 times or more. Other ratios of selenium to mercury are as follows: tilapia 68:1, cod 45:1, trout 30:1, mackerel 18:1, haddock 10:1, and swordfish/halibut 5:1. Only one fish, pilot whale, has more mercury than selenium, but few eat that. Thus it appears that the negative side of mercury in fish has been somewhat exaggerated because the abundant selenium keeps mercury at bay.

Eating smaller fish can also reduce mercury intake. Very large fish often contain more mercury than smaller ones like sardines. This is especially true when eating freshwater fish where selenium can be more variable. Of course, during pregnancy it is always good to be more cautious. The Institute of Medicine in the National Academy of Sciences states that pregnant women and young children can safely consume 12 ounces of seafood per week, but they should definitely avoid swordfish, shark, king mackerel, and tilefish.

A third worry-busting technique is to use capsules of fish oil. These supply lots of EPA and DHA and usually contain no mercury. You can get the mercury analysis from the manufacturer. But I prefer eating fish because of the abundance of other nutrients such as protein, vitamins and minerals, like selenium. Selenium itself plays an important role in preventing heart disease and some forms of cancer. So choose fish wisely, enjoy it, and let selenium do some of the worrying for you.

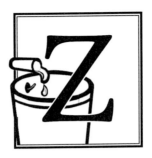

Zinc

Galvanize Your Health

The mineral zinc is essential to your health, but dietary deficiencies are on the increase. Vermonters in particular may be getting less nowadays in their foods. How can this be?

Zinc is probably best recognized as a treatment for metal, called galvanized metal, which slows the rusting process. Metals such as nails, water pipe, and sheet metal are dipped and coated in zinc. This prevents corrosion and greatly extends the metal's life. Would adequate dietary zinc extend your life expectancy too? Most likely! But you don't get coated with it because its biological functions are quite different.

Zinc functions primarily as part of hundreds of enzymes. Enzymes are cellular catalysts that speed up the rate of chemical reactions so that they happen much more quickly than they would in a laboratory test tube. There are thousands of enzymes in every cell in your body, and they operate continuously to keep cellular mechanisms working rapidly. A lot can go wrong if even one enzyme fails.

Although enzymes are made mainly of protein, some require zinc in their structure. If zinc is deficient many enzymes stop functioning. Among the hundreds of things they do, here are just a few. They are needed for skin growth, bone growth, sexual development, ability to taste, reproduction, embryonic development, blood formation, wound healing, and antibody production.

In a severe zinc deficiency, hair falls out and the skin appears rough and dark. Movie stars and cosmetologists sometimes promote zinc supplements to keep your skin young and beautiful. Sorry, it doesn't quite work that way although zinc is used in make-up powders, and in that sense you do coat yourself with zinc, but that doesn't make you healthier. (Yes, zinc oxide ointment is used with the treatment for skin infections, but that's not a nutritional effect.)

A curious case of zinc deficiency occurs in children. If severely deficient, they do not grow well and do not develop sexually. At 18-20 years of age they look like they are 10-12 years old. In girls, there is little breast development, lack of pubic hair, and immature body shape. In boys, they retain central baby fat, penises do not grow, and muscles remain immature. This occurs because zinc is needed for the production of sex hormones, and the deficiency is sometimes referred to as nutritional castration. Add zinc to the diet and normal development restarts within weeks. It's really quite remarkable. This had been seen a while back, mostly in the Middle East.

Although such severe zinc deficiencies are rare in the U.S., marginal or borderline deficiencies seem to be on the increase. We now know that dietary zinc is needed for our immune systems to function properly, and if deficient, the risk of getting a viral or bacterial disease increases. Because higher amounts of zinc are found in eyes and prostate glands, it's been proposed that zinc also prevents macular degeneration and prostate cancer. This is being tested, and we shall see. Zinc deficiency can also lead to diabetes, problems with taste and smell, poor wound healing, and sick babies.

Food, not supplements, is the best way to get zinc, and the best food source is meats. Next come unrefined grains. So a highly-refined diet lacking in meat is a culprit in causing borderline zinc deficiencies. Yes, vegetarians can especially be at risk. But because zinc leaches from galvanized metals into water and food, the increase in marginal deficiencies is also associated with the replacement of galvanized metals with plastic and other materials.

Maple syrup (the real stuff we Vermonters use) was once considered the most potent source of zinc. We use lots of it on pancakes, ice cream, and cereal. But now galvanized sap buckets are being replaced with plastic tubing and stainless steel is used in the construction of sap evaporators instead of galvanized sheet metal. Alas, our intake of zinc in Vermont is decreasing. So as technology changes, our health is becoming less and less galvanized – and that's the uncoated truth.

Healthy Holidays

Here as an added bonus are some *Musings* for the holidays.

Lyn

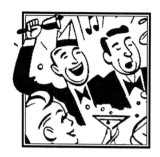

Happy New Year
Food Resolutions

It's that time of year again to think about New Year's resolutions. Have you made yours yet? Did they include any promises about the foods you would and wouldn't eat? Avoid chocolates and eat lots of spinach? But that gets boring and even a little irritating. In his hit book *In Defense of Food: An Eater's Manifesto,* Michael Pollan suggested that we in the United States concentrate too much on eating to prevent or cure diseases. Rather than eating to enjoy foods, we think of them as medicines. To quote him, the easiest formula about eating is this: "Eat food. Not too much. Mostly plants." That's ok, but I would suggest adding some protein in each meal.

Our discussion should end there, but if you're feeling guilty that you haven't made any New Year's resolutions yet, here are a few nutritional suggestions. Maybe you could pick one or two and feel you've done your job.

I resolve to...

– increase my intake of vitamin D. Here in Vermont this may require a vitamin supplement unless you travel to Florida each week. The latest evidence strongly suggests that a variety of problems including heart disease and multiple sclerosis are related to a deficiency of vitamin D. In addition, a deficiency of vitamin D readily occurs in the northern climates during winter.

– eat fish three times each week or take fish oil capsules. There are few other sources of the omega-3 fatty acids found in fish, and you could be deficient in them. Omega-3 fatty acids can improve mental performance, lower the risk of heart disease, and help in a variety of other ways.

– eat only unrefined grains. Refining removes most of the vitamins and minerals and leaves you with the starch that contains only energy, and this can make you fat.

– avoid eating sugary foods and too many fatty foods to help keep my weight in a reasonable range. Diabetes that accompanies obesity can shorten your life span and even cause blindness. And there is evidence that sugar can be addictive.

– avoid sugary soft drinks. They are loaded with calories and little else. The phosphorus in colas can cause bone problems, especially in growing children. Excess phosphorus may even play a role in kidney disease.

– drink water from the tap. Much of the bottled water sold in stores isn't as pure as claimed, and may have contaminants. Also, recycling the plastic bottles is creating a severe environmental problem.

– include green vegetables, especially leafy ones, in meals every day. They are good sources of vitamin K. Exciting new evidence shows that this vitamin plays a major role in reducing bone diseases and heart disease as well as helping with blood clotting. Also, vitamin K may be a major nutrient in controlling inflammation, a significant new concept that links inflammation with the cause of many diseases, including diabetes and cancer. And remember the American Cancer Society's recommendation to eat 1-2 servings of cruciferous vegetables daily to prevent cancer.

– be careful about depending on vitamin/mineral pills. Excess of vitamin A and folic acid from pills may cause a variety of problems such as weak bones and cancer. And, of course, many minerals such as iron and selenium in excess can be very dangerous.

– eat protein at breakfast, maybe even an egg, to help stay alert and awake during the morning. This really works. That popular breakfast of coffee and two donuts can be a killer. The sugar soon triggers fatigue and the caffeine stimulates the nervous system. What does bouncing between those opposing effects do to me all day long?

– worry less about some food components such as saturated fat and cholesterol. Half the people with heart disease have normal blood cholesterol levels. Some saturated fats lower blood cholesterol, and even act as antibacterial agents.

But on second thought, maybe making a whole bunch of New Year's resolutions isn't such a hot idea. They take a lot of mental energy and create stress. As a matter of fact, now I'm all stressed out just thinking about them. Maybe we should all just make one resolution. Let's take another piece of advice from Michael Pollan's writings. "Do not eat anything your grandmother would not recognize." There. Now that sounds like a good resolution and it's a lot easier. Besides it's kind of fun to think back to days of yesteryear and imagine what grandmother's old-fashioned meals looked like and imagine what she would not recognize today. Try it! You'll be in for a nice surprise.

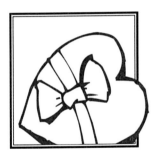

Valentine's Day
Chocolate ~ A Health Food

A box of chocolates on Valentine's Day may delight both the giver and recipient, although nutritionally it's not such a good idea. The candies are filled with sugar and fat. Yes, they may contain a nut or two and tiny amounts of coconut or other fruit. Nevertheless, they are still low on the nutrient scale. But wait! If we consider just the chocolate itself, we may be dealing with one of the best health foods available. Chocolate a health food? That sounds too good to be true.

Pure chocolate or cacao itself, the dark stuff surrounding all that sugar and fat in sweets, is loaded with many unusual substances (chemical compounds) that may be extremely beneficial for your health. But the chocolate must be dark and as unrefined as possible. Processed chocolate loses a lot of these benefits. So here is the yummy side of this story. Be careful reading this though, because I am a great fan of chocolate – a chocoholic – but I'll try not to be biased.

Why do people feel so good when eating chocolate? Could it be the sugar, even the fat? Not quite. There is scientific evidence that something in pure chocolate itself brings on this elation. Blood levels of a stress hormone called cortisol go down when dark chocolate is eaten. High blood levels of cortisol are partly responsible for common stressed-out feelings; therefore, the less cortisol, the better. But direct effects of chocolate on feelings of stress have not been measured. How much dark chocolate is needed? Nobody knows, but it may be as little as 0.35 oz (10 grams) per day, just a bite, and probably no more than 1.5 oz (40 grams) of minimally processed, real dark chocolate. That's about the size of a small Hershey bar and contains only 200 kilocalories.

Chocolate comes from cocoa beans, about the size of Brazil nuts, found within the fruit pods of a cacao tree. The strange cacao tree has the fruit pods growing out its trunk and big limbs – hanging there as if someone had pinned them on. A pod is 6-12 inches long, brownish, red-orange in color, and shaped like a football. The beans are fermented in the sun for a week, then roasted and ground, and the cocoa liquor (about 50 percent fat) is extracted. This end product is bitter so a little sugar is added and a powder formed. Essentially, that is what makes up candy bars and cocoa. Some chocolate bars contain 85 percent or more of the original cacao powder and this is real dark chocolate with all its health benefits. But frequently in making candy, especially milk chocolate, the cacao is much diluted. The more processed the chocolate, the less its healthful effects.

Besides lowering stress, dark chocolate is known to lower blood pressure; people in tropical countries who use lots of cacao powder in drinks or foods have significantly lower blood pressure. Cacao powder and dark chocolate are loaded with compounds called flavonols and antioxidants, which may slow the ravages of aging such as arthritis and heart disease. There is even evidence that pure chocolate prevents cancer and reduces inflammation, a process that is strongly correlated with many diseases.

It isn't easy to know how pure the dark chocolate you buy may be. The word "dark" stamped on foods made of chocolate may mean nothing. Look at the label and see if pure cocoa or cacao powders were used. The closer to the original cacao plant the better and any processing can destroy the flavonols and antioxidants; common alkaline treatment used to make cocoa for drinks is highly destructive. Several top companies, including Vermont's own Lake Champlain Chocolates, indicate the percent cocoa.

So don't shun the gift of chocolate as bad for your health. A bite or two of real dark chocolate can become part of a well-balanced diet. And, as I wrote this, what do you think I've been eating?

April Fools
Nutritionally Speaking

Did you survive April Fool's day? Did you wind up with a "kick me" note on your bottom? Did somebody tell you your clothes were ripped in an embarrassing place? Did anybody tell you something about nutrition and foods that wasn't true? Well, on the latter point, let's look at a few possible jokes in the nutrition realm.

Vitamin A is found in carrots. *April fool.* Plants do not contain vitamin A. Almost all vitamin A comes from foods of animal origin. Plants do contain large amounts of a yellow-colored pigment called beta-carotene that is converted to vitamin A in our intestines.

Vitamin D is a vitamin. *April fool.* It is not a vitamin but actually is a hormone. In an evolutionary sense, we were meant to get our vitamin D via exposure to sunlight and synthesis in the skin. A vitamin is something that must be supplied by food. If you are out in the sun for only a few minutes in the summer or in the tropics, you should not need Vitamin D in your diet.

Cholesterol is found in vegetable oils. *April fool.* There is no cholesterol in the plant kingdom. In spite of ads on television, vegetable oils such as corn and soybean never contained cholesterol at all. It's only produced by animals and therefore only found in foods of animal origin.

Eating sugar causes diabetes. *April fool.* Diabetes is either an autoimmune disease or caused by a virus (type 1), or related to obesity (type 2). Certainly eating too much sugar can make you obese and lead to diabetes, but so can almost any food. Too much sugar can make diabetes worse, but it is not a direct cause of this condition.

Avoid meat from chickens fed hormones. *April fool.* They don't exist, so you can't avoid them. Commercial chickens have not been fed nor injected with hormones since about the 1960s. It's illegal to do this. For a time the estrogen, diethylstilbestrol (DES), was injected into young broiler chickens to increase their fattiness – they were called caponettes. But because DES was associated with human cancer, this practice has been totally eliminated. So people who write stories and books proclaiming the danger of hormone-fed chickens are simply out-of-date.

You should drink eight glasses of water each day. *April fool.* Such a formal recommendation about drinking water has never existed. Yes, you can find it in textbooks, but it has no scientific origin. You should drink enough fluids that your urine is almost a clear color and not yellow: that's what is enough.

Sugar causes hyperactivity in children. *April fool.* Just the opposite. Too much sugar causes sleepiness in 99 percent of children and in adults too. Maybe that's why people drink coffee along with doughnuts in the morning.

Vitamin C prevents colds. *April fool.* There has never been a scientific study showing this. It may alleviate the symptoms a little, but that's all.

Babies fed early on solid foods sleep better. *April fool.* Starting babies on solid foods at three months or six months doesn't affect their subsequent sleeping habits.

Well, that's all of my April Fool's jokes for this edition. I hope you got a kick out of this list, and did not wind up with a note stuck to your bottom!

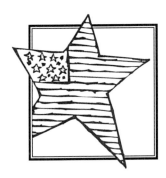

The Fourth Of July
Colorful Fireworks And Colorful Foods

On the Fourth of July, fireworks flash in the sky and display a variety of colors – reds, whites, blues, and many others –and make people happy. Foods are like fireworks. They too come in a variety of colors and can also make people happy. We are talking mainly about plant foods. The pigments that give plants their colors are called phytochemicals or phytonutrients, and they have a variety of beneficial effects on health. They may be responsible for preventing chronic diseases such as cancer, heart disease, arthritis, and evidence exists that they also affect our daily performance. It isn't sufficient anymore to talk about a "balanced diet" in terms of the simple food groups: grains, fruits, vegetables, meat, and milk. We also must think about balancing the colors of foods we eat.

Red – Studies in Italy suggest that men who eat lots of cooked tomatoes (yes, pizza and spaghetti) have less prostate cancer. A red pigment called lycopene may be responsible. Red sweet cherries have the most potent antioxidant properties of any fruit. Researchers at the University of Vermont have shown that cherry juice can improve muscle performance in athletes. And we have all heard of the "French Paradox" in which the French develop heart disease less frequently than we do in the U.S., despite eating foods loaded with creams and cheeses. This is mainly attributed to a substance in red wine, resveratrol (also found in peanuts). Other foods in this group are red cabbage and cranberries, and I'm sure you can think of many more.

White – Yes, even foods such as cauliflower, garlic, watercress, and onions have been reported to lower blood cholesterol, prevent tumors, and trigger detoxification in the liver. Some of the active substances are called allylic sulfides and flavonols, but knowing these names isn't important – just the food colors.

Blue and purple – For many years, blueberry growers have labeled this fruit as being loaded with antioxidants. Blackberries, Concord grapes, pomegranate, and almost any other blue-purple food you can think of are included here. I have even eaten blue potatoes! The bluish-purple anthocyanins in these foods not only may prevent chronic diseases, but they've been reported to improve mental performance such as memory decline associated with aging and even Alzheimer's disease.

Orange and yellow – This is the famous carotene group found in carrots and all other such colored plants: squash, yams, peaches, and cantaloupe. Beta-carotene is not only converted to vitamin A and prevents night blindness, but it has a marked anti-cancer effect. Two other substances in this category, lutein and zeaxanthin, have definitely been associated with preventing age-related macular degeneration.

Green – Chlorophyll gives the green color to plants, and little is known about its direct effects on health. However, eating green plants is extremely important for two reasons. The green color hides other underlying colors like the orange-yellow carotenes; we all see this when the leaves turn color in the fall. So most green plants are loaded with other colored phytonutrients as well as very powerful phytonutrients that do not lend a color to them. And if you read my previous piece on cruciferous vegetables, you'll remember that green members of the cabbage family – broccoli, kale, collard greens, Brussels sprouts and others – contain very powerful anti-cancer substances.

Brown – In discussions of food color and health, this group is often overlooked. This includes soybeans, whole grains, lentils, and other beans. The phytochemicals here are numerous, from lignans that may reduce the risk of cancer, to various sterols that may lower blood cholesterol, to hormones related to estrogens that can have beneficial effects on bone growth and cancer.

We haven't even covered the whole color spectrum here, but for now just remember to keep your food intake as varied in color as the fireworks that burst and boom on the Fourth of July.

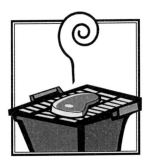

Labor Day
Cool Hand Luke And Cool Meats Too

The passing of actor Paul Newman brought to the limelight, once again, the concept of *cool*. Newman was certainly very cool in one of his most famous films, *Cool Hand Luke*. For this writer and many others, Newman was one of the greatest actors of all times, and he was also cool in movies such as *The Sting* and *The Hustler*.

But what does this have to do with Labor Day and September? Well, besides Paul Newman's cool, a different concept of cool occurred in September 2008. Although many people celebrate Labor Day, some people interested in food safety have been laboring for years to improve the labeling of imported foods. Did you ever wonder where many of your foods come from?

On September 30, 2008, a food labeling law known as Country of Origin Labeling (COOL) went into effect. Did you know this? If not, you might want to pay attention next time you are shopping. This law requires that most meats be labeled as to the country they come from. There was a law written under the 2002 USDA Farm Bill which required that certain fruits and vegetables and some fish be labeled as to country of origin. It originally included meats, but it was not enforced due to lobbying pressures, and the 2008 law is an attempt to make up for this deficit. For years, imported meats have had to be labeled aboard the ship in which they were being transported (called bin labeling) but once they landed in retail stores the law did not apply. But now they must be labeled in retail outlets. The meats included in the law are beef, pork, lamb, chicken, and goat; additionally, the law includes peanuts, macadamia nuts, pecans, and ginseng. But the law has one significant weakness. If the meat is at all processed, even cooked or tomato sauce added, the law does not apply. Therefore, only pure cuts of meat as found in retail stores would be required to have the labels. Restaurants, cafeterias, bars, and other food service organizations are exempt.

As you might suspect, there was strong pressure both for and against the law among food interest groups in the United States. People who produced foods locally in the U.S., such as cattle ranchers, strongly supported the bill, whereas those whose main business was importing foods opposed it. I would daresay the latter contingent had the more powerful lobbyists.

The classic example of concern about importing tainted meat occurred in 2004. The United States Department of Agriculture admitted that it had secretly allowed beef to be imported from Canada even though a 2003 outbreak of mad cow disease had occurred there and restrictions had been placed on beef imports.

Many people would like to know more about the foods they buy. Studies generally show that about two-thirds of the public do read a food label containing nutrition information; however, whether people act on this information or not is open to question. Studies of the effect of COOL labeling on food choices are rare. Nevertheless, the public should exert more pressure to promote labeling foods' origins. Especially so in light of the recent scares about contaminants such as melamine found in milk products made in China, which resulted in many babies becoming seriously sick. It's unfortunate that the rules in the 2008 Farm Bill are so weak. Nevertheless, from now on, like Paul Newman's characters, you may be cool when you put your hand on fresh meat in the supermarket, even if your name isn't Luke.

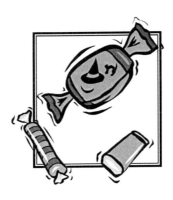

Halloween
Scary Sugar

After Halloween's trick or treating is over, the young ones have likely enjoyed an abundance of sugar that lasted all week. Is this a problem? How scary is sugar to one's health?

When I was young, we didn't have candy at Halloween because trick or treat hadn't been "invented." Only the trick part existed and Halloween was for pranks. Pranksters soaped windows, lit bonfires, and knocked on windows in the darkness of night. Wheelbarrows and porch chairs appeared on rooftops the next day.

But things are different now and in replacing Halloween tricks with sugary treats, perhaps we've created health problems. Sugar has been blamed for heart disease, obesity, cancer, behavioral problems, tooth decay, vitamin and mineral deficiencies, and many other diseases. Are these valid concerns?

The two principle negative effects of eating too much sugar are tooth decay and nutrient deficiencies. Sugar and sugary candies are known as "empty calorie" foods, meaning they supply nothing but energy – no nutrients at all – no vitamins, minerals, nor protein. To the extent that sugar supplies only calories, it can be blamed for a variety of mineral and vitamin deficiencies. For example, some children scamper off to school having eaten sugary breakfasts such as cookies and soft drinks, instead of healthy cereals and milk (yes, soda and cookie breakfasts do happen and that's scary). Such children can become deficient in vitamin B_6 (pyridoxine) and have learning problems. Vitamin B_6 is essential for the functioning of the nervous system. Adults eating too much sugar may be missing chromium in their diet; this could cause diabetes because chromium activates insulin. But in these cases it's wrong to blame sugar directly for these negative effects. Some sugar, eaten in a balanced diet, won't cause such problems. It's when nutrient-dense foods are replaced with sugar that there are unhealthy results.

Sticky sugar also leads to tooth decay, although good dental hygiene such as brushing on Halloween night can control this. For tooth decay to occur, three conditions must be met: there must be bacteria in the mouth, they must stick to the teeth, and they must have a simple food to convert to acid. Yes, tooth decay is a bacterial disease, and sticky candy meets the last two conditions. Without a doubt, sugar is a major culprit in tooth decay.

For many years, hyperactivity in children was blamed on sugar. This seemed obvious because children were "off the walls" in school the day after Halloween. It had to be the candy! The Feingold diet in the 1970s promoted the idea that food additives caused hyperactivity and sugar was dragged along with this theory. Later, several large studies showed the opposite effect: sugar probably causes sleepiness. Hyperactivity the day after Halloween is most likely the result of all the spooky excitement and lack of sleep the night before.

There is no evidence table sugar causes cancer, and the evidence that it causes heart disease is shaky. Another sugar, fructose, does elevate blood fat when eaten in the pure form and this can lead to heart disease, but this is a rare event. Fructose is normally found in combination with the sugar glucose, as in table sugar or high-fructose corn syrup (HFCS). In these forms, it doesn't seem to affect blood fat as much as fructose alone. But table sugar, fructose or not, is not the best thing to be eating.

Some top nutritionists have also blamed the fructose in HFCS for the obesity epidemic. They claim that the increase in childhood obesity, which started in the 1970s, parallels the increasing use of HFCS. But since fructose in HFCS appears in the same ratio to glucose as in common table sugar, why didn't table sugar cause this obesity years ago? Yes, eating too many calories from sugar can cause obesity, but too much fat or protein does the same thing. Be careful with such correlations, they can easily be misinterpreted and frequently don't mean much.

So yes, it is scary to think of all the possible relationships between sugar and bad health. But if a well-balanced diet is eaten along with just a little candy, and good dental hygiene is followed, the scariest part of sugar may disappear just like spooks after Halloween night.

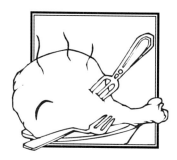

Thanksgiving Dinner
Sleepy Time Meal

Have you noticed what a wonderful warm, sleepy feeling comes along with Thanksgiving dinner? This is so common that as soon as the last morsel of turkey or dessert is gone the whole family may zonk out and nap, or conversely, they may take a brisk walk in the cold to wake up. A popular misconception is that the amino acid tryptophan in turkey meat is responsible for this occurrence. Yes, turkey does contain considerable tryptophan, and yes, tryptophan can make you sleepy. But there's a catch! The tryptophan must be consumed alone for the sleepy effect to occur: no other amino acids can be present. Turkey is high in protein and because all proteins contain 19 other amino acids in addition to tryptophan, ingesting tryptophan in the form of protein cannot make you sleepy. Research at MIT has proven this.

Tryptophan makes you sleepy only if it is converted into a neurotransmitter in the brain called serotonin. Serotonin's job is to relax the brain. Neurotransmitters are chemical substances that carry electrical charges from one brain cell to another – kind of like little ferry boats between brain cells. Of the 30 or so neurotransmitters in the brain, they can be divided into two groups: those that relax and those that excite. Fortunately, most of the time these two groups are in balance in the brain and we act normally. But if they get out of whack one way or the other, we may feel very relaxed or too excited. With too much tryptophan the balance is tipped toward relaxation and that sleepy feeling comes on. But if the other 19 amino acids are in the blood after a meal they prevent tryptophan from entering the brain and it can't be converted to serotonin. Hence that sleepy feeling will not occur. It's kind of like having 19 bullies standing on the street corner preventing the little kid from entering the store to spend his money. Tryptophan is bullied away from the brain by the other 19 amino acids found in turkey protein.

What then brings on that sleepy feeling as you push away from the Thanksgiving table? In part, it is created by the relaxed atmosphere of the holiday with family and friends. But in a significant way, it is likely due to the extra body heat produced as a result of eating so much food. Eating a lot produces extra heat and this makes us sleepy, just as a hot summer day makes us feel lethargic and lazy. In nutritional terms, this is called diet-induced thermogenesis or DIT. This is the heat resulting from the work of processing food and occurs in all animals. Metabolic mechanisms in the body speed up to handle and process the incoming food. The larger and quicker we eat a meal the greater this effect, and it persists for several hours. To the contrary, if we ate Thanksgiving dinner over several hours we might hardly notice the DIT. Also, protein and carbohydrates cause much more DIT than fat, so all that turkey and potato are major culprits. But keep in mind that all foods do this to varying degrees. So enjoy Thanksgiving dinner, and after the meal get rid of your DIT by going for a walk in the cold fresh air, or then again, just sleep it off if you wish.

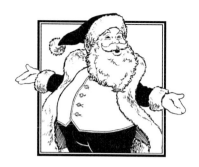

Christmas
Santa's Nutritional Gifts

I just got a note from Santa that he has some surprises for Vermonters this Christmas.

Cousin Vixen who lives near Lake Champlain is a dancer who eats lightly but needs a concentration of antioxidants to keep her overactive oxygen-burning muscles in shape and to prevent them from becoming damaged by free radicals. As Santa passes over Maine on his way here, he is getting a case of blueberries for her. He will combine them with some North Pole frozen red cherries, both of which are loaded with all those dark purple and red antioxidants.

Uncle Nicholas, who lives on Shelburne Point, loves spaghetti but always eats the stuff made from refined flour. Santa is going to place several boxes of whole-wheat spaghetti under his tree so he will get the increased fiber and the many nutrients in the bran that are usually lost during refining.

Aunt Mary, whose home is near the golf course, will receive several bags of whole-wheat flour. She loves making bread from highly-refined white flour, and the smell and taste are a treat at Christmas dinner. But she always complains of irregularity…Santa is going to help her with this one.

Poor sister Joy who moved to Jerusalem, Vermont, has bone problems and had lots of difficulties shopping for the family gifts. Santa has

81

round-trip airline tickets for her to travel to Florida in the winter months to get out in the sun and absorb all of that vitamin D. There's a bikini in her stocking. And because vitamin D is so deficient among Vermonters from October to April due to the low-lying sun, Santa intends to place a bottle of vitamin D pills in every Green Mountain stocking hung by the chimney with care. He said he would probably do this in Maine as well when he grabbed the blueberries (he gets his plums there too).

The Kringle family in the Northeast Kingdom has newborn twins. Santa is leaving infant formula because they are not being breastfed. It contains proper levels of omega-3 fatty acids from fish oil so their brains can grow rapidly and healthfully during the first year, and they will later be college stars at the University of Vermont. He made sure the formula was made locally. Santa is also planning to put a can of sardines in each Vermont stocking so that everybody will benefit from the omega-3 fatty acids. He knows it will help older Vermonters remember how many Christmases they have had and keep everybody else's heart in good shape (so they can shovel that three-foot Christmas snowstorm that is on its way).

Santa's elves sent out a message that Aunt Holly (the chocoholic who lives on the Canadian border), is going to get a year's supply of Lake Champlain Chocolate's darkest, purest chocolates and truffles. Unlike the white and milk chocolate she has in her purse all the time, these dark chocolates contain catechins or polyphenols that are sure to lower her blood pressure.

Of course, Uncle Gabriel is expected to get a case of Shelburne Vineyard's Coach Barn red wine, his favorite, which probably explains why he can eat all those creamy French foods and still have that great low cholesterol reading. Santa said he had sampled some of this and Mrs. Claus said his face now matched the color of his coat. And while he was thinking red, Santa said elderly Cousin Noel, who lives nearby and is pushing 80, is getting a case of tomato sauce loaded with that red pigment lycopene that keeps the prostate gland in check. Cousin Noel likes to make his own pizzas.

The six and seven-year-old Donners who live in the Green Mountains have been naughty because they drink cola at breakfast. They wrote Santa and said that if they got the train and dollhouse they wanted, he could also leave some cute, figure-eight shaped bottles of pomegranate juice, and they would be good for goodness sake and drink that at breakfast instead.

Well, this New Year is going to see many more healthy Vermonters because Santa helped and kept up with his nutritional reading and writing. It would be nice to meet him some day. Oh, and by the way, I always meant to ask Santa what on earth Rudolph eats to make his nose glow so red!

Lyn Carew's Favorite Christmas Party Mix

1¼ sticks (5 oz) butter

2 tablespoons Worcestershire sauce

1¼ teaspoon Lawry's Original Seasoned Salt

2 cups each (8 cups total) Wheat, Rice, Corn, Multibran Chex

2 cups mixed nuts (or 1½ cups mixed nuts, plus ½ cup whole cashews)

Cake pans 10 x 15 x 2" high

Melt butter in a pan in oven at 250° F. Remove and add Worcestershire sauce and Lawry's salt. Stir thoroughly with a metal spatula. Add Chex. Mix thoroughly with spatula to moisten all of the Chex. Add mixed nuts and mix again. Heat in oven at 250° F for four 15-minute cycles, removing the pan at each 15 minutes, and stirring the mix in oven for a total time of one hour.

Spread on brown paper (such as shopping bags) and let cool. Can be used immediately or frozen for several months.

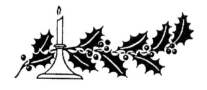

About The Author

Lyndon B. Carew, Jr. (Lyn) from Lynn Mass. received his doctoral education in nutrition, biochemistry, and endocrinology at Cornell University and pursued post-doctorate studies in muscular dystrophy there. His undergraduate studies were in genetics and poultry science at the University of Massachusetts, and prior to that he majored in agricultural leadership at the Essex Agricultural Institute, Hathorne, Massachusetts.

Since 1969, Carew has been Professor of Animal Science, and Professor of Nutrition and Food Sciences at the University of Vermont (UVM). During 42 years at UVM, Carew received every teaching award possible, including the most prestigious Kidder Award, and was named a Scholar in the Biological Sciences. He also received two national teaching awards from the USDA and from the *North American Colleges and Teachers of Agriculture.* In 1999, he was named Vermont Professor of the Year by the Carnegie Foundation for the Advancement of Teaching. Carew also has taught nutrition to industry, college, and school populations in Honduras, Ecuador, and Colombia, and to families in the remotest mountainous Andean regions. For years, he has had a close research association with the Zamorano Pan-American Agricultural School in Honduras.

His numerous scientific publications include topics in energy and protein metabolism, thyroid/mitochondrial metabolism, and fat, mineral, and amino acid physiology. He has researched a number of foods including soybeans and the velvet bean, a sustainable, subsistence crop used widely in underdeveloped countries.

Besides human nutrition, Carew has a deep knowledge of poultry nutrition and uses the chicken as the experimental model in much of his research. During five years in the 1960s, working with the Colombian Institute of Agriculture in South America, he directed development the National Poultry Program and Nutrition Laboratory as a member of the Rockefeller Foundation's team during the Green Revolution. He was popular there for his introduction of American-style barbecued chicken. Carew was director of Avian Drug Research for Hess and Clark in Ashland, Ohio in the 1960s.

He has engaged in numerous speaking and television presentations as well as written journalism articles. Carew served as President of the Vermont Nutrition Council for several years, increasing greatly its visibility during his tenure. He also authored the first ever college-level computerized course in nutrition in the early 1980s when the idea of computer-based instruction was dismissed by many.